Jace !

JACOB

THE Theory of Fat Loss

THE Theory of Fat Loss

A New Paradigm for Exercise

Timothy J. Ward

Edited by David D. Aguilar
Contributions by Jake Skrabacz

Copyright 2010 © by Timothy Ward. All Rights Reserved.

No portion of this book may be used, reproduced, or transmitted in any form or by any means, electronic or mechanical, including photocopy, fax, recording, or any information storage and retrieval system by anyone but the purchaser or reviewer for their own personal use. This book may not be reproduced in any form without the express written permission of Timothy Ward except in the case of a reviewer who wishes to quote brief passages for the sake of a review written for inclusion in a magazine, paper, journal, or website- and these cases require written approval from Timothy Ward prior to publication.

Disclaimer

The information in this book is for educational purposes only. There is an inherent risk assumed by any participant with any form of physical activity or change in diet. Those wishing or planning to change their diets or participate in an exercise program should check with their physician prior to initiating such an activity. Anyone participating in such an activity should understand the dangers of doing so regardless of whether the activity is performed correctly or incorrectly. The author of this book assumes no liability for any adverse outcomes. This is purely an educational book to guide those who are already proficient with the demands of any such activities.

While the author has made every effort to provide accurate Internet addresses at the time of publication, the author does not assume any responsibility for errors or changes that occur after publication. Furthermore, the author does not have any control over and does not assume any responsibility for third-party websites or their content.

ISBN-13:
978-1456389109

ISBN-10:
1456389106

ACKNOWLEDGMENTS

First and foremost, I have to thank my family. Without my parents, Bernard and Cecilia Ward, I never would have been born. Without my brother Benjamin Ward, I never would have had somebody to look up to. Without my sister Melissa Ward telling me how small and weak I was growing up, I never would have gotten into the field of fitness and sports performance.

Thanks to my friends, especially David Aguilar, Bobby Kenney, and Tom Perron. You've been my best friends since 4th grade, and I appreciate everything you've ever done for me. I'd also like to thank Jake Skrabacz. Our weekly conversations about training drastically improved every aspect of this book. Thanks as well to all my clients, especially the females. Without you, I never would have had that "a-ha!" moment that led to the concepts detailed throughout this book.

My professional development is due largely to studying the work of other fitness and nutrition professionals, several who do not even know who I am. In no particular order, I would like to thank Mike Robertson, Bill Hartman, Eric Cressey, Mike Boyle, Alwyn Cosgrove, John Berardi, Mike Roussell, and Nate Green.

I would also like to thank Diane Pitts, for when I was her student, she always treated me like a colleague and a professional, not a subordinate.

Finally, I would like to thank Pat Rigsby, Nick Berry, and Brian Grasso. You are extremely successful and powerful businessmen, yet you stay grounded and always take the time to help me out and listen to my thoughts and ideas.

For Gramps because he has always believed that I could accomplish anything that I put my mind to.

Contents

Foreword by Jake Skrabacz   *xi*
Introduction   *1*

Part 1. Fat Loss Constructs

Unit 1: The Theory of Absolute Intensity
Chapter 1: The Absolute Intensity Theory of Fat Loss   *8*
Chapter 2: Case Study 1- Absolute vs. Relative Intensity   *11*
Chapter 3: Objectifying Absolute Intensity   *15*
Chapter 4: Force, Work, and Power   *17*
Chapter 5: Time (and Volume)   *21*
Chapter 6: Exercise Selection and Cardiovascular Load   *23*
Chapter 7: Relative Intensity   *26*
Chapter 8: Special Topic 1- Morbid Obesity   *28*

Unit 2: The Limiting Factor Theory
Chapter 9: Cae Study 2- The Limiting Factor   *32*
Chapter 10: The Limits   *35*
Chapter 11: Capacity Limits and the Tradeoff Concept   *38*
Chapter 12: Functional Limits   *42*
Chapter 13: Knowledge Limit Tradeoffs   *45*
Chapter 14: Coordination Limit Tradeoffs   *47*
Chapter 15: Postural and Injury Limit Tradeoffs   *50*
Chapter 16: Time Limits and Tradeoffs   *52*
Chapter 17: Programming Limits   *53*
Chapter 18: Special Topic 2- Aerobics and the Energy Systems   *55*

Part 2: Fat Loss Practical

Unit 3: The Construct Compound
Chapter 19: The Theory of Fat Loss   *64*
Chapter 20: Fat Loss Programming System   *66*
Chapter 21: Assessment and Programming Forms   *71*
Chapter 22: Special Topic 3- Women   *76*
Chapter 23: Case Study 3- Using the System   *78*
Chapter 24 : Dedicated Fat Loss Programming   *84*

Unit 4: Nutrition and Other Factors for Fat Loss Success
Chapter 25: Nutrition Basics   *90*
Chapter 26: Eating- When, What, Why?   *92*
Chapter 27: Choosing Foods   *95*
Chapter 28: Diet Consistency   *98*
Chapter 29: Sleep   *101*
Chapter 30: Attitude and Environment   *102*
Chapter 31: Goals   *105*

Conclusion   *107*

The Appendices
Appendix A: Posture   *112*
Appendix B: Mechanism of Soft-Tissue Injuries   *115*
Appendix C: The Warm-up   *117*
Appendix D: Youth Obesity   *120*

Foreword

If you're reading this book, titled *The Theory of Fat Loss*, I'm going to take a wild stab in the dark and say that you're *not* sporting a midsection that deserves its own nickname and that will single-handedly earn you a spot on the next big reality TV show. In the spirit of speculation, I'm also going to go way out on a limb here and say you may not have the body of your dreams *in spite* of trying <u>everything</u>. Luckily, you've picked up exactly the right book. Not only will you learn why *everything* didn't work, but also you'll find the something that *does.*

I was there. I had tried everything. I was 21 years old and could not remember any day in my life that I was happy with what I saw in the mirror. I played all the sports while growing up. I starting lifting weights in high school in addition to varsity swimming, cross-country, and track. When I wasn't out running 8 miles per day, I was swimming 250 laps per day. When I wasn't doing either of these I was in the weight room 6 days per week. Yet I never had anything close to visible abs. Even when I hit the lowest weight I've ever been since puberty during my third and final cross-country season, I never dropped below 18% body fat. So I ran and ran and ran. I ran myself through shin splints. I ran myself into a stress-fracture. The frustration finally caught up with me and my running career ended as soon as I stepped foot in the ER. That day, I *accepted* that I just was born with a certain "body type" and that nothing was going to change my body composition. The best I could do was stay in shape. I coasted through college at 21% body fat. At least I was consistent!

How does this relate to *you*? Perhaps you're thinking, "21%! I'd love to be there by the end of next year!" Or perhaps you're thinking, "Why's this fatty writing the foreword of a book on fat loss?" Either way, we both know what it's like not to be happy with our body composition. In fact, I'll venture to say that both of us know what it's like not to even be content. I know the path you've been on, but more importantly I know the new path you've begun by picking up *The Theory of Fat Loss*. It's the one where you tap into *physical* and *mental* potential you never knew you had, and you get the results you want. How do I know? I began 2010 at 21% body fat.

I am ending it at 9%. Why? Because I met Tim Ward. I believed in the training paradigm he has presented in this book, and today I am the leanest, strongest, fastest, most flexible, and most muscular I've ever been. I'm not a fitness professional. I'm not an athlete. I'm just a graduate student trying to juggle solid dieting and training with my pursuit of a PhD.

"Of course… another fat loss success story, but that doesn't mean this all will work for *me*," you may think. And why wouldn't you?! You've tried everything already, and in spite of people seeing results all around you, you never have. Well, this isn't just another program, and it isn't another theory of fat loss; this is *THE* theory of fat loss. You'll see what I mean after reading it. You'll also stop believing that nothing will work for you. With the skills you will learn here, fat loss will no longer be that insurmountable task perpetually haunting your to-do list with each passing assortment of New Year's resolutions. It will just be something you get done—an exciting ever-challenging part of your routine.

The best part is, you don't have to wait. After reading this book, nothing will be delaying your journey to a head-turning physique anymore. I get the feeling that after reading this book, you will feel like it was created just for you—the one who has tried *everything*. That's because it was.

-Jake (Sausage Link) Skrabacz

Introduction

The title of this book is quite bold: *THE Theory of Fat Loss*. Perhaps it is just this author's ego being put on full display, but after finishing this book, you will be able to decide for yourself whether the information was indeed as valuable as claimed.

Assuredly, it is expected that by word of mouth several people will come to hear the title and basic premise of this book and dismiss it or even argue vehemently against it without ever taking the time to read it themselves. This is okay, as it cannot be avoided. It is simply human nature to take as many shortcuts as possible when forming our opinions. Thus backlash, as unwarranted as it may be, is both welcome and anticipated.

Of course, the title of this book is not meant to be taken literally. Like any concept in fitness, it has its limits, and there are probably hundreds of flaws and loopholes to be found in it. But the point of the title is not so much to make this book out to be the Bible as much as it is to provoke thought. This book will indeed be far reaching even if it is not as all encompassing as it is meant to sound.

In the fitness industry, old terms get thrown around in new ways every single day. In fact, because there are so few new ideas in the world of fat loss that have any relevance, it is amazing to me that people keep buying new books on the subject. How many fat loss books are written every year? If they work so well, then why do new books keep coming out? Human physiology has changed so little in the past thousand years that it is very doubtful that something that worked last year isn't going to work as well as something new that came out this year.

The theory this book will expand upon is meant to be what this author believes is a new paradigm for fat loss programming. It is a distinct concept. It is a novel way of thinking about and looking at fat loss.

The bread and butter of this fat loss paradigm is a combination of two constructs: *the theory of absolute intensity* and *the limiting factor theory*. There is no doubt that many other fitness professionals have thought of variations of each of these individual theories. Likewise, after reading the chapters on these theories, you will find them to be so intuitively obvious that you will wonder whether either of them is new at all. In fact, neither is new. They have been thought of thousands of times and applied (whether deliberately or by accident) millions of times.

It is the unique combination and description of the two constructs that comprise the new paradigm, this *Theory of Fat Loss*.

But really, how new is this going to be? As already stated, human physiology has changed very little and what worked last year is still going to work this year. New books are just old ideas packaged in shiny wrapping and given fresh titles.

It is impossible to calculate how many effective and ineffective fat loss programs have ever been written. This book, this theory, is new not because of what it is but because of what it is not. It is not another program. It is not a step by step guide telling you how and when to exercise. It is not a manual telling you to do this and that and not to do these and those.

It is *the underlying theory of exercise programming for fat loss*. Rather than being a little blue pill one can swallow to magically shed off 20 pounds through blind faith and direction following, this is an educational book designed to enlighten and empower you to be able to create, examine, and critique any fat loss program **in the context of your own personal needs and abilities**. It will teach you to filter out all the half-truths, all the gimmicks, and all the false advertisements designed to prey on your weaknesses and insecurities. It will free you to decide for yourself where to go and what to do. Your only limits will be your imagination and self-commitment.

People say that a book is a snapshot of the time in which it was written. By the time a book gets published and read, it is typically years outdated. This author believes that this theory (not necessarily the book and its examples, however) will be timeless. Fads come and go. Philosophies change with the seasons. The best professionals continue to improve their programming. This theory, as deeply rooted as it is, will perhaps hold true through it all.

In addition, I believe this is one of the first books of its kind that is meant to reach both the lay person who is serious about exercise and the avid fitness professional desiring to learn more in an ongoing quest to perfect the craft. It is both simple enough for anyone to understand and profound enough to provoke thought in the most accomplished fitness authorities.

In its purest form, a theory can sprout, grow, and expand in an infinite number of ways. As such, it is this author's hope that this theory will be used to launch millions of new ideas, millions of new programs, and millions of new success stories. So without further ado, let's begin.

Author's Commentary- This book will make use of commentary boxes. These comments and musings, which will be loosely related to the subject being described, are to be taken as the author's personal thoughts or opinions (and you may choose to agree or disagree at your own convenience). These comment boxes may offer flavor, personality, humor, perspective, or this author's personal anecdotes. Some chapters will have a lot of commentary (and may even have more commentary than non-commentary) and others will have little to none. If you do not care to read the author's commentary, feel free to skip over these boxes. He will not be offended.

The best fiction book I've ever read is *Anthem* by Ayn Rand. When asked why I like this book so much, I always respond, "The chapters were short." Honestly, I can't even remember what the book was about, but I do remember thoroughly enjoying it because many of the chapters were less than 3 pages long. Because of this, I read the entire book in one night. When you are reading a good book but have other important things to do, do you ever say to yourself, "Oh, I'll just finish this chapter. There are only 3 pages left"? I did this with *Anthem* about 15 times. Before I knew it, the book was over.

Likewise, my favorite textbook when I was in physical therapy school was *Essentials of Musculoskeletal Care*. Why? Instead of having a 150-page continuous chapter entitled "shoulder" or "knee" like most books, this book had big "shoulder" or "knee" units that were hundreds of pages long. However, each individual condition or injury started on a new page like it was its own individual chapter and was described for only a few pages. Psychologically, it is much easier to read 3 pages at a time than it is try to make sense of 150 continuous pages of nonsense.

Therefore, I have decided to keep the chapters in this book as short as possible. That way, if you get bored with a topic (and you probably won't), you at least know it will be over soon. Similarly, if you are interested in continuing (and you will be) but have some other matters to attend to, perhaps you will just say to yourself, "Oh, I can read one more chapter. It's only 2 more pages!"

Part 1: Fat Loss Constructs

The Theory of Fat Loss is composed of two separate constructs that become truly potent when integrated. Part 1 will explore the intricacies of these two constructs in detail

Unit 1:
The Theory of Absolute Intensity

This unit will draw a picture of the first construct,
The Theory of Absolute Intensity

Chapter 1

The Absolute Intensity Theory of Fat Loss

Have you ever known anybody (and maybe you or one of your friends fits this description) that has tried "absolutely everything" but cannot seem to lose weight or keep it off? This is the person that lifts weights twice a week, runs three times a week, attends fitness classes every night, and is very health-food conscious, showing initial progress but then ultimately ending up right back at stage 1 the moment the routine is thrown off for as little as a few days.

Likewise, have you ever seen a media story about a professional athlete in his offseason that reports that he is not in shape or has let himself go? Do you ever wonder how it is that this athlete, a month later, can report to training camp looking like a world beater?

How is it that your Average Joe or Plain Jane can't seem to do anything right to cut body fat but an elite athlete can go from twenty to twelve percent body fat in only a month?

The trend among human beings is to walk the path of least resistance. In the modern era, there is a lot of talk about genetics. So now, to justify one's own failures or shortcomings, one must simply strike up a conversation about genetics. Since few people in the non-scientific population actually know the slightest thing about genetics, most will simply agree with whatever is said about it in order to appear informed and save face.

This can be exemplified by the following scenario:

Mike and Joe are watching football on Sunday and start up a conversation.
Mike: Ya' hear Perkins from Carolina lost 20 pounds the month before the season started?
Joe: Yeah, its ridiculous. I've been trying to lose weight for so long. I've tried everything.
Mike: You haven't tried *everything*. Whatever he did to lose 20, you haven't done.
Joe: That's the thing. I got his workout from a magazine and followed it to a T. It kicked my

butt, but I only lost 2 pounds! I'm tellin' you! It's genetics. He's only in the pros because he was born to be in the pros. That's why he can lose weight like its nothin'. Regular guys like you and me just can't compete with that. There's nothing we can do.
Mike: You're probably right.

Unfortunately, and I hate to admit it, my mother uses this excuse for herself and for my brother regularly. (The ironic thing is that my brother needs no excuses and knows that he has the ability to lose weight if he chooses to put forth the effort, and he willingly admits it.) No amount of logic can change her mind. Perhaps I should try a more personal approach. Rather than arguing with her, I can have a heart to heart conversation with her about what she has tried and what she hasn't tried and really find out about her goals, letting her know that I am here for her if she decides she wants to take the first step. At the same time, I can really get to know her as a person and not just as my mother. On second thought, I'll just spend a few months writing this book. Then when it is in circulation I can say to her, "It is foolish to argue with me. I WROTE THE BOOK ON FAT LOSS!"

Anyway, I am absolutely not saying that genetics have nothing to do with one's ability to cut body fat. I just find that the idea is well overblown and is used as an excuse to a much greater extent than its actual effect. Anyone can cut fat, no matter their genetic makeup.

In most situations, making it to the elite level requires years of structured and dedicated training. To make it to professional football, for example, an athlete typically plays 4 years of high school and then 4 years of college. No high school or college football team exists that does not require the athlete to partake in a strength and conditioning program. (If such a football team exists, they would not win very many games). By the time an athlete makes it to pro football, he has at least 8 years of training experience. That training continues throughout his entire pro career.

Depending upon what time of year it is, an athlete is going to focus on a certain training goal. For example, a football player may be in a training phase where he is going to get bigger, stronger, more explosive, more agile, or better conditioned. Training phases such as these are cyclical, and an athlete will *very* rarely focus on the same goal year round.

For example, imagine that Mike Football, a Junior at State University, just finished up his competitive season and is going into the offseason. His biggest weakness is that he lacks size. So, for the first 12 weeks of his offseason he trains to put on some mass. He increases his caloric intake to complement his training. Satisfied with his improvements, he works on strength and power for the next 8 weeks. Because he is training to get stronger, he continues ingesting vast quantities of food. After this phase is completed, Mike is bigger and stronger than ever, but he is also up to 16% body fat from the five months of eating so much. He has one month left before his season begins and he needs to get in "game shape." This final month of his offseason is spent on conditioning or "getting in shape." Mike gets his body fat to 8% and enters his Senior year the biggest, strongest, and leanest he has ever been.

On the other end of the spectrum, we have Joe Chill, a 28 year-old accountant, who likes to kick back and relax year round. He realizes one day that his wife is no longer attacking him nightly with the same fervor she did during the first few years of their marriage. He looks down and sees his enormous gut, so he decides that he needs to lose weight and lose it fast. After a month of blood, sweat, and tears, Joe (and his wife) is unsatisfied and gives up, discouraged because he tried so hard and accomplished so little.

Again, how is it that Mike could make so much progress in a month when Joe could not make a dent in his physique? By now, you probably are thinking, "It's obvious. Mike trained hard for 6 months (and probably for years before that), so when it came time for him to lose weight, he was able to train a lot harder and handle a lot more than Joe. I didn't need to buy this book for you to tell me that."

Exactly.

You have just deciphered the *Theory of Absolute Intensity*, which states: *The greater the absolute intensity one can achieve with training, the greater the fat loss result will be.*

Chapter 2

Case Study 1- Absolute vs. Relative Intensity

On New Year's Day every year, tens of thousands of people make a fat loss resolution. "This year, I'm going to lose 30 pounds," or, "My husband won't be able to keep his hands off me by the end of this year because I'm going to look like a model."

Let's say Max makes a 30 pound fat loss resolution this year. He is serious this time, and he writes out a goal to help him start out the year with a bang. "I will lose 10 pounds in January." After doing so, he asks himself, "How do I go about losing ten pounds in one month?" Max just finished reading the first chapter of this book and recalls the theory of absolute intensity. "The greater the absolute intensity..."

Max's plan is thus to train as hard as possible all month. He refuses to end a workout if he is not sweating profusely, short of breath, and ready to vomit. By the end of January, he has completed 24 workouts and is down 11 pounds. Max is happy with his result and gets compliments from his wife and all his friends. They ask him how he did it. He says smugly, "hard work- training every day so intensely that I want to throw up."

February rolls around and Max is a little burned out from January. He decides that since he already lost 11 pounds (which is more than 1/3 of his original goal in only 1/12 of the year), he can take it easy this month. He spends the entire month doing some light lifting and about 30 minutes of steady state cardio most days of the week. He loses 4 pounds in February.

Motivated by the fact that he lost 15 pounds in only two months, he thinks to himself, "This fat loss thing is way easier than everyone makes it out to be. I'm going to lose these last 15 pounds this month!" March looks much like January. The only difference is that Max is in better shape than he was when he started so he makes his workouts a little more intense than before. Motivated Max again completes 24 vomit-inducing workouts.

He steps on the scale in the gym on March 31st and has lost 2 pounds. "What! This scale must be broken!" Convinced that the scale lied to him, he weighs himself at home. This second fiendish scale confirms the worst: he has lost only 2 pounds. Although Max is disappointed, he refuses to give up. He thinks that maybe he just did not pick the right exercises. In April, he goes back to his gym and hires a trainer to write and coach him through a one month fat loss program. The exercises in April are new and difficult and Max feels like dying after each training session. Midway through the month, after experiencing a whole new world of hurt, Max says to himself, "This must be what that book meant by *absolute intensity*."

Unfortunately for Max, April is the cruellest month. He again lost only 2 pounds, and there is no way he could endure another brutal month like April again in May. He begins to understand what people mean when they say losing weight is hard. May, therefore, becomes another month of light lifting and steady state cardio. "I'll just maintain my weight this month, then in June I can train hard again."

The career of a typical personal trainer is about 2 years. That's it. This is particularly true in those big commercial gyms and health clubs where the focus is "SELL SELL SELL" and not trainer education and lifelong learning. Most clubs have personal training packages that offer something like an assessment, an assessment and 10 sessions, or a 6 week _____ program designed to do _____ and _____ in just 6 weeks guaranteed. Of course, any good trainer knows that a short term program is useless if not in the context of a long term program, but that fact is lost on trainers who work for gyms that are designed only to make money. Any trainer can help a newcomer put on muscle or lose 10 pounds of fat in 6 weeks. When someone is new to training, absolutely everything will work. This fact is often exploited for large profits and is the reason why short term programs will always be around.

Most trainers get into the industry for all the right reasons- to help people achieve their goals. The one's that lead successful careers are dedicated to lifelong learning. They are *fitness professionals*. They read every book they can get their hands on. They buy information products from the most successful people in the industry. They read research journals on strength and conditioning and exercise physiology. They attend seminars whenever they are being offered. They talk to other trainers. They visit other gyms. While it is certainly possible that a *fitness professional* can work for a commercial gym, he or she will often leave as soon as possible to start a private business or join forces to work with other like-minded individuals that truly are passionate about what they do.

If you are a trainer, ask yourself this: **Are you making your clients better, or are you just making them tired?**

If you have hired a trainer, ask yourself this: **Is my trainer making me better, or is my trainer just making me tired?**

Any workout should be done to help achieve a short term goal that is in the context of a long term goal. If a workout seems like a random collection of exercises thrown together for no other reason than to make you tired (like some of the "insane" and "extreme" done for you DVD products on the market), then it is probably of limited use.

What seemed like a great maintenance plan at the time resulted in Max gaining 6 pounds. June and July, Max's last ditch effort for training intensely, result in a 5 pound loss. Max gives up in August and stops training. He gains 10 pounds, and he does not even care anymore. If we add all that up, we get a net loss of 8 pounds in 8 months. It probably will not get better come September. What went wrong?

The reason for this chapter is to clearly demonstrate the difference between *absolute intensity* and *relative intensity*.

The Theory of Absolute Intensity states that the greater the absolute intensity one can achieve with training, the greater the fat loss result will be. This is not to be interpreted as "train as hard as you can right now and you will lose fat."

If you are an untrained, sedentary individual, almost any amount of exercise will leave you tired and out of breath. If you can only squat 100 pounds, then squatting 85 pounds ten times will leave you tired and out of breath. If you have been in a coma for 15 years and then wake up and try to walk up a staircase, you will be tired and out of breath. The point is that you can always find something that is difficult for you to do. If something is difficult for you to do, it is intense for *you*. That is, the *relative intensity* is high. *Absolute intensity* is something entirely different and cannot and should not be estimated based on how you feel during or after a workout.

This means that to lose fat effectively, your number one goal should be to increase your *intensity capacity*.

In Max's case, he failed because he never spent time "getting in shape to lose weight," if that makes sense. Rather, he jumped right into training at his highest relative intensity which left him a burned out failure. If he would have spent the time increasing his intensity capacity instead of trying to take a shortcut and lose fat fast, he would have had great long term success.

I just mentioned that absolute intensity has nothing to do with how you feel during or after a workout.

Most people very incorrectly assume that they had a good workout if one or more of the following is true:

1. They are sweating a lot
2. They have been breathing heavily or are short of breath.

Case Study 1- Absolute vs. Relative Intensity

3. They have muscles that are "burning"
4. They have a great muscle "pump"
5. They are sore the next day

These are very subjective measures and none of them have anything to do with anything. In fact, if those are measures of how great a workout is, then why don't you try some of the following three workouts?*

1. Put on a sauna suit, and then go eat dinner in a sauna. You'll sweat a lot, and thus your "consumption workout" will be more intense.
2. Chemically induce a heart attack. Shortness of breath is a classic sign of myocardial infarction and is also a great indicator that you are having a good workout. For less dire consequences, substitute a panic attack.
3. Have your friend punch you repeatedly in the thigh, or better yet, have your friend stab you in the thigh. I guarantee soreness the next day. Great workout, bro.

*In today's litigious world, I have to go ahead and tell you that I was being sarcastic. Do not do any of the three "workouts" I just suggested. They are all terrible ideas. Thank you.

Anyway, different workouts designed for different goals feel completely differently. It is the hardest thing for people to understand. Not all workouts are designed to make you feel like keeling over, nor should they be. In fact, I would (and I have) instantly discredit a personal trainer if he created a workout entitled "plyometrics" that was an hour long and that was meant for extreme fat loss. Anybody who studies or coaches performance enhancement knows exactly what I'm talking about and will probably laugh at the irony.

As I continue with this book, I'll also be sure to mention how, based on my own subjective experience, different programs are supposed to feel.

Absolute intensity is directly related to calorie expenditure (both during the workout and for the hours and days after the workout ends), and that is why something that is more absolutely intense than something else is better for fat loss. When two people compare their workouts, the workout that had the greater absolute intensity resulted in the greater calorie expenditure. Even if somebody in great shape is not even remotely tired after a workout, he or she still could have had a much more calorie intensive workout than someone who was throwing up or gasping for air. Again, how somebody feels during or right after a workout is a measure of *relative intensity* and has little to do with fat loss.

Chapter 3

Objectifying Absolute Intensity

A good theory should be objectively measurable in some way. The rest of this unit will break down the *intensity factors-* the components of any single workout that are used to objectively determine absolute intensity. On an absolute scale, which is more intense:

1. Deadlifting 500 pounds or deadlifting 100 pounds?
2. Squatting 100 pounds or half-squatting 100 pounds?
3. Jumping 36 inches or jumping 24 inches?
4. Running at 10 mph for 30 minutes or running at 10 mph for 2 minutes?
5. Spending 3 seconds lowering a barbell to your chest or spending 1 second lowering it?
6. Resting 1 minute between sets of an exercise or resting 3 minutes between sets?
7. Performing 5 full body exercises or performing 5 biceps isolation exercises?
8. Achieving a heart rate of 180 or achieving a heart rate of 120?
9. Training as hard as you can or training half as hard as you can?

Hopefully it is very obvious that the first choice in every pairing is absolutely more intense than the second choice. Those pairings highlight nine different intensity factors. They are:

1. Strength (or Force)
2. Range of Motion
3. Power
4. Workout Duration (or Volume, depending on how you look at it)
5. Time Under Tension
6. Rest Time
7. Exercise Selection
8. Cardiovascular Load
9. Relative Intensity

You may be able to think of other factors that play a role in determining absolute exercise intensity. If so, more power to you. This book will analyze the nine listed above.

I purposely chose examples that are intuitively obvious and are free of confounding variables or controversy. Notice I did not compare things such as steady state cardio (running, cycling, elliptical training, etc.) and interval training or steady state cardio and resistance training.

While it is my personal opinion that steady state cardio is immensely inferior per unit time to both interval training and resistance training **for fat loss** (the absolute intensity that can be achieved with steady state cardio is simply not that impressive), it is not a simple one sentence explanation to describe which is more intense because there are too many variables.

Then again, if you ever have observed men and women in commercial gyms "training," you would understand why people think running for an hour burns more calories and results in greater fat loss than resistance training.

Seriously. Your stereotypical female who gets lost in the free weights section of the gym because someone told her that lifting weights burns more fat than her favorite exercise, elliptical running, will pick up a dumbbell that weighs around 5 pounds and will perform curls, triceps kickbacks, shoulder presses, front raises, lateral raises, and rows... all for 3 sets of 15... because light weights and high reps are for people that "want to tone." On the flip side, your typical male will spend his entire week performing 37 different variations of bench press, biceps curls, and crunches and will completely forget that he has 2 legs and a back.

If you disregard those people, however, you will find that a good resistance training and interval training program (or a freaky blend of both) will always trump a properly programmed steady state cardio program. If you refuse to believe me, that's fine. Just don't complain when your mother and her formerly fat friend look better than you because they took me seriously. It's not my fault the industry has lied to you for the last 40 years. Anyway, after finishing this book, it will all make sense to you, and you'll wonder both why and how everyone else can still be so ignorant of this fact.

Chapter 4

Force, Work, and Power

Force, work, and power are three interrelated terms you will find in any introductory physics textbook. They will be defined below using both physics and practical terms.

Force is equal to the product of mass and acceleration. In exercise, the product of mass and acceleration is equivalent to "weight." For the purpose of this book, "strength" will be used instead of the word "force". In practical terms, a person's strength is equivalent to the maximum weight he can lift. It is pretty obvious that **a greater absolute intensity is required to lift heavy weights than is needed to lift light weights**.

Mechanical work is equal to the product of force and distance. For exercise, think about "work" as "range of motion under tension." Even simple "range of motion" is far more practical. If you keep "weight" as a constant, **moving an object through a greater range of motion requires a greater absolute intensity**. The same is true for an exercise like towing a sled (except now instead of "weight" we have "friction"). If you keep the loading the same, more work is done when the sled is moved farther.

Power is equal to the quotient of work and time. If you define power in terms of exercise, you get *power = strength x range of motion / contraction time*. In other words, someone with great power is someone that is both strong and able to complete tasks rapidly. As an example, picture someone jumping three feet into the air and then that same person jumping two feet into the air. Jumping three feet in the air required a greater force and less time spent in contact with the ground (less time under tension) when compared to jumping only two feet. Therefore, greater absolute intensity was required for this person to jump three feet into the air. **With great power comes great absolute intensity**.

... and great responsibility. Ain't that right, Spidey?

In review, greater strength, greater range of motion, and greater power are equivalent to greater absolute intensity, and you know by now that greater absolute intensity results in greater fat loss.

At this point, you may be wondering something.

You might have noticed that one of the *intensity factors* listed in the previous chapter is "time under tension." You probably figured out that more time under tension equals greater absolute intensity. With power, it seems as though you are trying to minimize time under tension. Are these two intensity factors contradictory? How do you determine which intensity factor is more important?

It doesn't really matter. With every exercise or exercise program, there is going to be a tradeoff or a limiting factor. For example, you might be able to lift a heavy weight 3 times or a light weight 100 times. When trying to cut body fat, which do you choose? The real answer here is that it is impossible to say out of context. I would need to know several other things before answering your question, such as your body weight, your maximum strength, your cardiovascular endurance, your muscular endurance, and what the rest of your workout program looks like, to name a few. In fact, the whole purpose of Unit 2 is to address potential limits.

The purpose of Unit 1 is to describe the *theory of absolute intensity* all by itself, not to describe it as if it were the only important piece of the *theory of fat loss*. There is another whole construct that we have yet to explore at this point. So, all I am suggesting is that you don't get ahead of yourself. Make sure you have all the pieces of the puzzle first before you try putting it together. Otherwise, you might end up with a picture that is missing someone's head.

The question now becomes, "What does this mean for me and my training?"

Range of motion is the simplest to address. When you are training for fat loss, go through the full range of motion, or even a greater than full range of motion (provided it is safe). If you are doing pushups, for example, you can prop yourself on your fists, go down until your chest touches the ground, and then come all the way up pushing your shoulder blades forward and apart as far as they go. That is considered a greater range of motion than your basic pushup. Another example is performing a reverse lunge off a box. The elevation requires that you step down lower than you normally would if you started on even ground. For exercises that you cannot modify to increase the range of motion safely, simply perform them through the full range of motion.

Again, there are going to be strength and endurance tradeoffs if you go through a greater range of motion, but just keep those concerns in the back of your head until the time comes.

It is also a fantastic fat loss idea to spend time increasing your maximum strength. You know that greater strength means greater absolute intensity, and you know this because it makes intuitive sense. It takes quite a bit more energy (calories) for your body to produce a lot of something than a little of something. What you might not have thought of is the effect of strength training on your body after the workout is completed.

Whenever you train, you are inflicting damage on your muscles. The heavier you lift, the more damage you do to them. It takes much longer and requires more of your body's resources to recover from a workout that causes a lot of muscle damage than a workout that causes just a little muscle damage. Of course, your bones, nervous system, and endocrine system also have a lot more recovering to do after a strength workout, so do not forget about them either. All in all, your body will burn a tremendous number of calories in the days following a strength training session than it normally would. The same is true when training for power.

Maximum strength just might be the single most important *intensity factor* that I am covering in this book. If you get one thing and one thing only out of this book, make it this:

Strength is the single greatest determinant of how effective a fat loss program will be.

Of course, this is my personal opinion, and I'm sure plenty of people will disagree with me. Even so, it would be foolish for anybody to say that maximum strength is not an important factor in fat loss. Likewise, it would be equally foolish to say that strength is the only important factor in fat loss.

A former client of mine who made a ridiculous body transformation in the period of one year was once asked the following question by a fellow gym-goer:

"You look amazing. What's your secret? Did you do low weights and high reps, or what?"
"No... I did HIGH weights and high reps."

Some secret.

Of course, saying that strength and power training is only useful because it significantly aids in short term fat loss would be selling it short. The truth is that strength training will give you the greatest long term return of any type of training. Unlike endurance training or any type of conditioning where the physiological effects only last a couple of weeks without continued maintenance, the effects of strength training are far more resistant to degradation. Years without any kind of dedicated training at all can pass by and strength will remain largely unchanged. Even with degradation, strength seems to return very quickly upon resumption of strength training activities.

What does this mean for fat loss? This means that even if you gain weight again, you won't need to spend as much time preparing for another long period of training to lose it if you properly strength trained the first time. Your intensity capacity will remain elevated from your previous training, and you will therefore achieve results much more rapidly the second time around!

This book is not about strength and power training, and if you need help with this type of training, check out the resources page of this book's website. You can find it at:

http://thetheoryoffatloss.blogspot.com/

If you never have strength trained before, keep in mind that strength training feels far different from any type of training you might be used to. Strength workouts that I design (other coaches may do things completely differently) will **not** leave you out of breath or fatigued (at least in the traditional "I couldn't pick up 5 pounds right now if I tried" sense of the word). Your muscles probably won't be on fire and you likely won't get any type of "pump."

Between sets of the same exercise, you will get full or near full recovery. However, each work set of every strength exercise will require intense focus (if it doesn't, you aren't loaded up enough) and each rep will be difficult to perform. After the strength sets, you might feel like you can and should be doing a lot more. In fact, some of my clients have told me after a strength workout that they don't feel like they did anything at all! Ignore this feeling, and trust in your program. If you do, you will make rapid gains in strength and will be stronger than you ever thought possible (and that will result in greater fat loss potential down the road). If you don't, you will be disappointed with your lack of results.

Typically, people realize how difficult strength training is on their bodies a few weeks into a strength program. You might notice you are walking a little funny, that you can't jump as high or perform in activities as well, or that there is simply something a little awkward about the way you move or feel. Trust me when I say that you'll know what I'm talking about when you get there (and when it happens, it is probably safe to say you need to take a deload week).

Chapter 5

Time (and Volume)

The next three *intensity factors* this book will cover are time variables. The first is *workout duration*; the second is *time under tension*, and the third is *rest time*. All three of these factors are very simple to understand, and thus not much time or space will be spent describing them.

Workout duration is simply the length of one's workout or training session. **A longer time spent training at a consistent intensity is more absolutely intense than a shorter time spent training.** Picture a runner going 8 miles an hour for 10 minutes. Then picture that same runner going 8 miles an hour for 20 minutes. Twenty minutes running is obviously more intense than 10 minutes of running if speed is held constant. Another simple example to wrap your mind around is the concept of activity levels. Even though daily activity level is not necessarily equated with "working out," it is still valuable to compare them. If you have a desk job, go home after work and watch TV for 4 hours, and then go to bed, you lead a sedentary lifestyle. Your activity level is low. If you, on the other hand, are a caddy and spend your day walking around a golf course, your activity level is fairly high. You are active for many hours a day (in other words, you have a long workout duration), and thus your absolute intensity is higher.

A different way to think about this (and in actuality, this is probably a better way to think about it) is by considering training *volume* as the important intensity factor in place of *workout duration*. The person that runs for twenty minutes as opposed to ten minutes simply took more steps. The duration of the workout is simply a byproduct of increased volume. **A more voluminous workout is more absolutely intense than a shorter workout.**

Two important notes:

1. I don't advocate running as an effective form of fat loss training for reasons that will be described in Chapter 18.

2. Using *volume* as opposed to *duration* avoids term ambiguity. Have you ever known a guy that spends two hours in the gym every day and doesn't actually do anything but check out the female talent? Basically, he'll go to the gym and perform a set or two of bench press, take a 30 minute "creep out all the girls" break, and then perform a few sets of "curls for the girls" before looking at himself in the mirror for ten minutes. Two hours pass by, and he's only done a total of about 6 sets of exercise. Don't be that guy. *Duration* only makes sense as an intensity factor if time is actually spent training at a consistent level. *Volume* will always describe how much one gets accomplished training.

Time under tension refers to the amount of time your muscles are active during a certain exercise or activity. **A longer time under tension is more absolutely intense than a shorter time under tension**. Imagine performing a squat exercise with a loaded barbell. Perform 10 repetitions. Now, imagine performing ten repetitions but taking five seconds between repetitions just holding the bar. The second situation was more intense than the first because you spent more time stabilizing your body under that bar. Another way to think about this is by imagining slow repetitions. Instead of performing 10 repetitions normally, perform 10 repetitions where you spend 3 seconds in the downward movement phase of the squat. That extra time spent lowering the bar makes for a more intense set of exercise.

Rest time refers to the amount of time taken between sets of exercise. Assuming you hold everything else constant, **a shorter rest time is more absolutely intense than a longer rest time**. Although *relative intensity* is not a good predictor of fat loss, you will find that you have a greater *relative intensity* with shorter rest times. You can tell by paying attention to how tired your body feels. Since you only are comparing shorter rest times to longer rest times (and holding everything else constant), it is safe to say that having a greater *relative intensity* with shorter rest times also means that you are exercising at a greater *absolute intensity* by shortening your rest times. As a practical example, imagine that your workout has you performing three sets of twelve deadlifts at 135 pounds. It would be fairly easy to take three minutes of rest between sets. It would be fairly difficult to take only 15 seconds of rest between sets. Your heart, lungs, and muscles will let you know which one is more difficult if you do not know already.

This is a point worth reiterating. Although I just said that a greater relative intensity does mean a greater absolute intensity, fight the urge to use relative intensity (or how difficult your workout is *to you*) as a measure of how difficult your workout actually is absolutely. If you are still having trouble with this concept, feel free to re-read Chapter 2. That, or wait patiently until you get to Chapter 7.

Chapter 6

Exercise Selection and Cardiovascular Load

Exercise selection and *cardiovascular load* are better described as combinations of other intensity factors rather than stand-alone variables. For purposes of clarity, however, they will be defined as if they were independent.

The exercises you choose to perform for any given workout go a long way in determining how intense that workout will be. **The total amount of full body muscle force needed to perform an exercise, the range of motion of the exercise, and the amount of time it takes to perform the exercise all go into determining the intensity of an exercise**. If we have 100 pounds, a biceps curl will be less intense than a leg press which will be less intense than a squat which will be less intense than an overhead squat. Similarly a lunge will be less intense than a lunge + shoulder press combination exercise. Get the idea?

There are plenty of different ways to increase absolute intensity with exercise selection. Here are just a few examples:

1. Performing multi-joint exercises (bench press) over single-joint exercises (triceps extension)
2. Performing combination exercises (two exercises blended into one compound movement)
3. Complexing (performing a group of exercises sequentially without putting the weight down)
4. Choosing explosive exercises (jumps, throws, Olympic lifts, sprints)
5. Performing exercises that require greater full body stability (such as Turkish get-ups, standing exercises, single-leg and single-arm exercises, overhead exercises, offloaded exercises, bottoms-up kettlebell presses, etc.)
6. Any combination of the above or others not listed here.

By this point, you can probably see why exercise selection is more of a combination *intensity factor*. Rather than describing this abstractly, here is a concrete example:

John wants to perform an exercise that will be extremely intense, so he decides on a complex that will include five repetitions each of single-leg Romanian deadlifts, bent-over rows, hang cleans, and front squats to push press at 135 pounds. This one massive exercise will be a blend of many intensity factors including great strength and power, a large range of motion (the bar is going to travel from near the ground to over head throughout the course of the exercise), a very long time under tension, zero rest time between exercises, and as a result of all this, a phenomenal cardiovascular load (described below).

> I could have addressed this in Unit 2, but I feel like it is more important to say it right now.
>
> There are plenty of studies showing that unstable surface training (like performing squats on a stability ball) activates a greater amount of muscle mass than traditional movements. Are these "training methods" more absolutely intense than traditional methods and thus better for fat loss? Not necessarily. One of the biggest factors for absolute intensity is how much force is produced when training. With unstable surface training (especially for the lower body), your loading takes a HUGE hit. For any exercise, you have muscles that will act as "prime movers" and muscles that will act as "stabilizers." For an exercise that requires a lot of stability, your stabilizers will be very active to prevent you from falling over. Your prime movers, on the other hand, will not be used anywhere near their maximum capacity because your stabilizers will likely have already reached their capacity limit (see Unit 2) for stabilizing you. Any extra loading would make you fall over, not make you recruit more prime mover muscle. An exercise that requires little stability will allow for maximum prime mover recruitment (or maximal loading). Extremely stable activities, such as "training" with machines, are the wrong way to go as well because they require far too little recruitment of those stabilizer muscles.
>
> The key is being able to perform exercises that allow you to get the greatest force production out of your prime movers AND your stabilizers. Those exercises should theoretically lead to the greatest fat loss because they are the most intense.

Cardiovascular load is determined by how much blood your body needs and how fast your body needs it. A couple things go into determining this: your body mass and your current level of activity. If you have a great body mass (either you are extremely muscular, carry excess adipose tissue, or a combination of both), you simply have a greater amount of tissue that needs blood. If you are training, you are draining your muscles' resources, and you need blood delivered quickly to replenish those resources. Basically, the bigger you are and the more active you are, the more blood you need delivered to sustain you. At this point, it should probably go without saying that **a greater cardiovascular load is more absolutely intense than a lesser cardiovascular load.**

The possible misconception that a greater heart rate is equal to a greater cardiovascular load is bound to come up in someone's head at some time or another. This is similar to the *absolute vs. relative intensity* discussion. If you want a great measure of relative intensity, you can take your heart rate. A higher heart rate at any given time is going to be more intense than a lesser heart rate. That is true. However, heart rate is not a valuable predictor of cardiovascular load, and therefore, it is not a valuable predictor of absolute intensity. Anybody who has read even the most basic book about exercise can tell you that your heart gets stronger as you get into better shape. This means that it pumps more blood per beat. So, if you are a trained individual (see Chapter 18 for a discussion of cardiac output development), your heart rate will be lower with the same amount of exercise than if you were not a trained individual.

Chapter 7

Relative Intensity

Relative Intensity is in fact an intensity factor. You already are very familiar with what it is, and possible confusion regarding relative intensity has already been addressed in Chapters 2, 5, and 6. Like exercise selection and cardiovascular load, *relative intensity* is a combination factor and not a stand alone concept. It is influenced by absolutely every other intensity factor.

1. Strength
2. Range of Motion
3. Power
4. Volume
5. Time Under Tension
6. Rest Time
7. Exercise Selection
8. Cardiovascular Load

Do those seem familiar? It is important to note that each and every *absolute intensity factor* listed above can also be thought of as a *relative intensity factor.* If you lift heavier weights during any individual workout, that workout is harder than it would have been had you done everything exactly the same but chosen lighter weights. You can apply the same concept to all the other factors.

What is the difference? Although you can make any **individual** workout extremely difficult for **you** by working at your own maximum capacity, it will not necessarily mean a thing for fat loss. As I have reinforced in the preceding chapters, fat loss results from operating at a high level of absolute intensity, regardless of how such a workout makes you feel. In order to perform at the kind of level conducive to fat loss, you may need to spend a few months improving your abilities.

Each individual workout should be designed to increase your *intensity capacity*. That means you should train to be stronger, more powerful, more conditioned, etc. In doing so, you can greatly increase the *absolute intensity* with which you train.

It is far more fruitful to push yourself to the brink of passing out when doing so will actually yield the results that you want. **A high relative intensity is more absolutely intense than a low relative intensity**. So when you and your body are finally ready to attack fat loss with everything you have, be sure to go all out.

Is it possible to be so well trained and to have an intensity capacity that is so great that you can train at a low relative intensity and still cut fat? I guess that theoretically it is possible, but you probably won't find anybody who can do this. First of all, the training required to reach that point would probably be more than enough to burn fat. So, if somebody reached that point, he or she would likely not have much fat left to lose. I suppose that if a person that didn't like me very much was training just to spite me, he could go ahead and train really hard to get to this point while at the same time ingesting 20,000 Calories a day so he stayed fat. Then, he could train at a low relative intensity (but still a very high absolute intensity) and cut his Calorie ingestion to normal levels and prove me wrong. I hope this person exists.

Anyway, when you are ready for a dedicated fat loss phase, how should you be prepared to feel during and after your workout? The optimal workout for fat loss is going to be at the greatest absolute intensity possible (meaning that the relative intensity should also be as high as possible). I'm not saying you should throw up after your workout or not be able to catch your breath for 30 minutes afterward, but if this does happen, you know that you pushed yourself to the limit. Basically, an all-in fat loss workout is going to make you not want to move (or maybe unable to move) for a while after you are done with it.

Chapter 8

Special Topic 1- Morbid Obesity

Within any theoretical framework you will find peculiarities that do not seem to fit within it. Throughout this book, the message so far has been to spend time increasing your intensity capacity before you try to participate in a dedicated "fat loss" phase of training. It is this author's sentiment, however, that those people who have a lot of fat to lose can jump right into fat loss training.

Before explaining why this is, it is important to clarify what is meant by "people who have a lot of fat to lose." Contrary to 90% of college girls' own beliefs that they are "fat," this does not often apply to them. What this chapter is referring to is people who need to lose fat for reasons that may not have anything to do with aesthetics. So, this chapter does not apply to a young woman who wants to "look good" for Halloween or maybe not even to a 220 pound, six foot tall male who wants to lose 20 pounds so he can dunk a basketball again. This chapter is solely referring to those that, for some sort of health reason, need to lose fat NOW.

If somebody is over 100 pounds overweight, it is (in most cases, anyway) safe to say that that person has not been living an active lifestyle and is much more than just a little "out of shape." Now, for your typical "out of shape" individual, it would probably be a good idea to spend time training as discussed throughout this book before trying to cut fat.

Is it different for the population described in this chapter? If these people, who are far more out of shape than your average couch potato, can jump right into fat loss, does this mean that there is a way for anyone to avoid a dedicated training program to increase one's intensity capacity before attempting a fat loss phase of programming? No.

Here's why. Those who are morbidly obese operate at a high absolute intensity whenever they do anything involving their bodies. Think about strength as an intensity factor. If you weigh 300 pounds and can stand and walk, your legs are likely tremendously stronger than somebody who weighs 160 pounds. Think about volume. Volume is a product of sets, reps, and load. If you weigh 300 pounds, your loading for any activity that involves moving yourself is going to be great, and thus any training you do is going to have a higher volume per repetition or set. Think about time under tension and rest time. If you weigh 200 pounds, try putting on a 100 pound weight vest and carrying it around all day without ever taking it off. The 300 pound person is constantly under great tension and essentially has no rest time when moving about. Finally, think about cardiovascular load. Part of what determines cardiovascular load is body mass. If you have a lot of body mass, your heart needs to work hard to get blood to all that mass.

Of course, this does not mean that a very heavy person can just start out training as hard as possible. That is going to result in serious medical complications. All it means is that this person is not going to need a dedicated strength or power phase of training. This person is not going to need to learn how to train through a great range of motion or learn how to perform exercises that activate the greatest total muscle mass. All that is irrelevant. What this person needs is a better diet and **any** type of exercise that gets him or her safely moving about because the absolute intensity will already be high.

Unit 2: The Limiting Factor Theory

This unit will paint a portrait of the second construct, The Limiting Factor Theory

Chapter 9

Case Study 2- The Limiting Factor

Chris hired a trainer to help him put on some muscle mass. The trainer, after assessing Chris, decided to put him on an undulating periodization hypertrophy program with 4 full-body workouts per week. Here is a copy of a part of the first phase of the program:

Workout A (Workouts 1, 3, 5)	Sets/Reps	Load	Rest	Sets/Reps	Load	Rest	Sets/Reps	Load	Rest
A Trap-Bar Deadlift	4x8		90	3x12		60	5x5		120
B1 TRX Rows	4x8		0	3x12		0	5x5		0
B2 Dumbbell Press	4x8		60	3x12		45	5x5		90
C1 Corner Barbell Anti-Rotation	2x8		0	2x10		0	2x12		0
C2 Side Plank	2x20s		60	2x25s		60	2x30s		60

Workout B (Workouts 2, 4, 6)	Sets/Reps	Load	Rest	Sets/Reps	Load	Rest	Sets/Reps	Load	Rest
A TRX RearFootElevated SplitSquat	5x5		120	4x8		60	3x12		60
B1 Pullups (TRX Assist as needed)	5x5		0	4x8		0	3x12		0
B2 Dumbbell Shoulder Press	5x5		90	4x8		60	3x12		45
C Ab-Wheel Rollouts	3x5	Levels:	60	3x8	Levels:	60	3x12	Levels:	60

Just to make sure you understand how this workout is performed, here is a description. Chris had two workouts (A and B) and 3 different set/rep schemes for each workout (4x8, 5x5, 3x12) for a total of 6 different workouts. He would perform workout "A" on Mondays and Thursdays, and he would perform workout "B" on Tuesdays and Fridays. If workout "A" was a 4x8 workout, then the next day's "B" would be a 5x5. The next "A" would then be a 3x12 and the next "B" would be a 4x8, and so on and so forth. Each workout had the following elements:

A. Lower Body Lift (bilateral for workout "A" and unilateral for workout "B")
B1. Upper Body Pull (horizontal pull for "A" and vertical pull for "B")
B2. Upper Body Push (horizontal push for "A" and vertical push for "B")
C#. Core (anti-rotation for "A" and anti-flexion for "B")

The load Chris chose was dependent upon the set/rep scheme for the day. Thus his 5x5 days were heavier than his 4x8 days which were heavier than his 3x12 days. His lower body lift was always done independently. This means that he would perform, for example, all of his trap-bar deadlift sets and reps before moving on to his upper body lifts. So, on his 4x8 day, he would complete a set of deadlifts, rest for 90 seconds, and then complete another set. This would continue until he completed all 4 sets. His upper body lifts were supersetted. That means he would perform "B1" and then immediately move on to perform "B2" before taking any rest time.

Anyway, after a couple weeks on this program, Chris had progressed nicely in exercise technique, loading, activity tolerance, and physical appearance. He was also figuring out just how hard he could push himself each workout. On one of his last 5x5 workouts in this phase, he decided to use a load for his deadlifts that was heavier than he had ever tried before. He got about 2 good reps before his form started to deteriorate. His **limit** for that lift was muscular. His back extensors could not maintain enough stiffness to safely complete all 5 reps of the deadlift under that amount of loading.

On his last 3x12 workout, Chris used a greater load for his single leg lift than he had ever used previously for a 3x12 workout, completed more unassisted pullups than he had before, and used a greater load for his dumbbell shoulder presses than he had ever used before. Because this was a 3x12 day, Chris's muscles had little problem with the loading because he was used to far greater loads on both his 5x5 and his 4x8 training days. Despite this, Chris could not physically complete the workout. He was completely exhausted by his second set of upper body lifts. His heart was pounding and he was breathing rapidly. He told his trainer that his muscles had plenty left to complete the last set but that he just could not catch his breath. Although the load was something his muscles could handle, the combination of that increased loading with the higher reps and lower rest time of this 3x12 workout caused another system to reach its limit. His **limit** during that workout was cardiovascular and respiratory.

It always bothers me when people say you need to do "cardio" to burn fat or lose weight. Of course you need "cardio" to burn fat. You need "cardio" for everything you do. If you don't have a heart to pump blood, you won't be alive for very long. When people say you need to do "cardio" they are more often than not incorrectly referring to some sort of steady state training. Steady state exercise is very limited in practical applications, yet it is rampant in our culture to the point of absurdity. There is nothing magical about running at the same pace for 5 miles. If you like running AND can stay healthy doing it (which most people can't), by all means, do it. Just don't try to tell me it is the best thing for your heart and health and physique because it is far from it. If you want to get in a great workout for your heart, there is a plethora of other options. How do you know what's good and what isn't? Take your heart rate.

I interviewed a former client of mine for an article I wrote about fat loss, and he illustrated this exact point to me. Here is what he said:

After just completing 2 sets of 20 alternating sets between front squat to push press and step ups (20 each leg!) with little enough rest that it amounted to well over a negative work to rest ratio, I was sitting there gasping, dripping sweat and waiting to gain some level of coherence after just completing 120 reps in like 7-8 min. One of my gym acquaintances picked this particular moment to come up and ask me, "Oh hey, I was wondering...what do you do for CARDIO?" I said, "I don't know. What do YOU do for resistance training?"

In exercise, a limit is anything that delays or prevents someone from reaching his goals. In the context of this book, *a limit is anything that negatively impacts one's ability to achieve or maintain a great(er) absolute intensity.*

You might have realized from reading Chris's example that there is never just one limit. In fact, there are always multiple potential limits during a workout. The first limit you reach just ends up being the most important one. Along these same lines, limits are not relegated to just individual exercises or workouts. You can find limits anywhere. There can be limits in your short or long-term program, in your diet (you may have heard that you cannot out-train a bad diet), or elsewhere in your life outside of training.

Of course, the focus of this book so far has been solely on exercise, and it will continue to be; therefore, the limiting factor theory and the limits that will be described will only emphasize exercise. It is important to note, however, that diet is a HUGE part of fat loss, as is your state of mind and training environment. Unit 4 will address some of these additional topics.

The Limiting Factor Theory, in terms of fat loss, states: *Within any fat loss program exist multiple potential limits that can inhibit one's ability to achieve success.*

Chapter 10

The Limits

In the previous chapter, Chris was used to introduce the concept of limits. If you recall, his two limits were muscular and cardiorespiratory. Those limits are directly related to the intensity factors described in Unit 1, and they will be referred to as *capacity limits*.

There are other limits directly related to your fat loss training. Of particular importance are the *functional limits*. A functional limit is something that prevents a person from being able to move effectively or efficiently. The functional limits that will be described in this book are exercise knowledge, coordination, posture, and injury.

Programming limits describe factors related to an exercise, individual workout, short term program, or long term program that limit one's progress towards a fat loss goal. *Time limits* describe factors that limit one's time to train. These can be daily time limits (having only 1 hour a day to train) or more global time limits (having a wedding two months from now)

In summary, the four categories of limits that will be described in this book are:

1. Capacity Limits
2. Functional Limits
3. Time Limits
4. Programming Limits

For those of you that like origin stories, you might be interested in knowing where the two constructs, *the theory of absolute intensity* and *the limiting factor theory*, came from. You'll be happy to know that they were born directly from observations in the gym and that I did not just make them up.

Below is an excerpt from the original piece I wrote that eventually led to me writing this book. You'll immediately identify some obvious similarities between this piece and what you have already read. Also keep in mind that my audience for this piece was college-aged individuals (and mostly men), so the language I used may be a little more colorful than you might like.

I have recently taken on a bunch of female clients. They are the reason I decided to write this today. You see, women, more so than men, feel that if they don't breathe really heavily during their workouts that they aren't effective. This is absolutely not true, of course, but if I can give them a really cardiovascularly demanding workout at the same time I am getting them to achieve strength goals, then I am making them feel better psychologically, which translates into better workouts and better compliance. As I've heard many times before, "Psychology beats physiology every time."

Before taking on this recent group of women, I had almost exclusively trained men. The obvious thing about untrained men as compared to untrained women is that untrained men are much stronger in practically all lifts. I usually have a 3x12 day with very little rest between sets for my beginner males. They always hate it because they can't use really heavy weights and by the end, they are so out of breath that they can hardly finish their workouts. They always feel that they can lift the weight, but their whole system is telling them to stop because they can't breathe.

You see, the limiting factor is not their musculoskeletal systems, it is their cardiovascular systems. When I hear people break resistance training and cardio into separate categories and say that resistance training isn't cardio, I get pissed off. I always think, "You just try one of my workouts, a-hole."

But something funny happened when I started training girls. Remember, untrained women are weaker than untrained men... and it's not even close. Most guys can easily trap bar deadlift 200 pounds on their first attempt (even if their form is crap). Most adult women can't get 100... and if they can, they do it, say it's too heavy, and don't want to attempt more. It is even more dramatic for the upper body. Few girls can do a single pushup or pullup.

I knew all this, of course, but what I found out in the first few weeks of training girls is that they just don't get very tired weight training like guys do. I can program 3x12 for girls and they do their workouts just fine. They don't breathe very heavily. They don't swear up and down because they are gasping for air. They do, however, struggle to finish their sets sometimes because their muscles give out.

I was telling these girls that they'd be getting a great cardio workout from resistance training with me, but they weren't. I didn't know what was going on. Then I thought that maybe the cardiovascular response isn't based on relative workload. Maybe it is based on absolute workload. Shoulder pressing 10 pound dumbbells alternated with some TRX rows (inclined to meet their level of strength) for 3 sets of 12 just wasn't all that cardiovascularly demanding apparently. You see, their limiting factor was not their cardiovascular systems at all. It was their musculoskeletal systems.

What led me to this absolute workload theory was a combination of my girls not getting very tired with their initial workouts and my personal lifting experience. You see, I regularly trap bar deadlift around 300 pounds. I can get about 10 reps at that load. Usually my muscles give out around then. I'm also always out of breath, but it usually doesn't limit me. My muscles do. However, sometimes I throw on 225 pounds for fun to do as many as I can. You'd think that if i could do 300 for 10 reps, I'd be able to get 225 for a lot more reps than 10. I can't. I can get to about 14, and then I lose my wind and put the weight down. My muscles are always fine.

Theory: Heavier absolute loads, not relative loads, determine cardiovascular demand.

Let's apply some numbers. Let's say Mary can deadlift 100 pounds plus her body weight of 100 pounds for a 1 rep max. We assign her 70 pounds to deadlift for 4 sets of 8. That's 85% of her total strength going into each rep.

Let's compare that to John, who can deadlift 400 pounds plus his body weight of 200 pounds for a 1 RM. We assign him 310 pounds for 4 sets of 8. That's 85% of his strength going into each rep.

I'd bet money that John's heart and lungs get worked far more than Mary's. More calories go into lifting that much more weight. More muscle mass is recruited. It only makes sense that heavier absolute loads are harder on the cardiovascular system than lighter ones.

Chapter 11

Capacity Limits and the Tradeoff Concept

Since the entire first unit was all about the intensity factors and increasing intensity capacity, you should be very familiar with them. How do these things come into play as limits? Well, if you recall, the whole purpose of increasing intensity capacity is to be able to maximize the absolute intensity you can train with during a workout so you can burn more fat. Of course, if you only have a small intensity capacity, you are going to reach your *capacity limit* very quickly during a training session. This, of course, is what you want to avoid when training for fat loss.

The capacity limits are:

1. Local muscular strength and power limits (how much one can lift or how much power one can produce)
1a. Local muscular endurance limits ("reproducible" strength, how long a muscle can last in terms of sets and repetitions or time under tension at a given load and with a given rest time)
2. Cardiovascular and respiratory limits (aka cardiorespiratory limits- how long the whole body can sustain training at a given intensity)

The most important thing to understand about cardiorespiratory limits that most people will forget or ignore when they assess themselves is that the limit is defined by the level of intensity and the type of training being performed (if you like highlighting in your books, this might be a good paragraph to highlight). **There is no such thing as a global cardiorespiratory limit.** By this I mean that a person might be fully capable of running 5 miles at a 6-minutes per mile pace but might be completely destroyed by a light weight training circuit. Likewise (and this is probably more important from a strength training standpoint), a person might not reach any cardiorespiratory limit while training with one load, but when that load is increased, the limit might be discovered. The following example might help clarify this if you are confused.

One of my clients was about to perform a circuit of three exercises for five sets of six repetitions each. She had performed this workout several times before and never reached a point where she was gasping for air or needed to take more rest time than was listed in her program. I decided that we should increase the load of just one of the exercises by five pounds to make it a little more challenging. To my surprise, that five pounds made a world of difference. She almost couldn't handle it, and it wasn't her muscles that were the problem. Her form during her sets was fine. Her heart and lungs just couldn't keep up. We hit her cardiorespiratory limit with those extra five pounds.

With that said, I expect that some people will probably want to argue that I should use another term for cardiorespiratory limits or define a new category like "energy system limits" because the description I use now isn't 100% accurate or clear. To those people I say, "No." The concept is more important than the science or the physiology or the semantics. I'm keeping it simple. For a discussion of energy systems, please see Chapter 18.

Switching gears, one note I'd like to make about strength limits is that they can also come from small muscle groups while performing high intensity exercises. I know I have said earlier in this book that the exercises that are the best for fat loss are exercises that work the most muscle, but this is not always true if a small muscle group is holding back the load you can use. For example, even if your legs can handle a 300 pound deadlift for 10 reps, what happens if you can't grip the bar for that long? Your wrists are your strength limit. What if you want to do a combination lunge and shoulder press for 20 reps per leg. Would it possibly be better to just superset the exercises instead if your shoulders could not handle a worthy load?

Capacity limits will apply to individual exercises and workouts. You may be able to estimate what your capacity limits are if you train fairly regularly. Other times, you hit a capacity limit during a workout. If you reach a capacity limit during a workout, that exercise or workout will come to an end **unless** you can get under that limit again. The only way to do that is to decrease your training intensity in some way or another. For example, imagine you are trying to perform a front squat for 3 sets of 15 repetitions at 135 pounds and are supposed to be taking only 30 seconds of rest between sets. After the first set, you realize that there is no way you can do another set at that load 30 seconds from now. You reached a capacity limit. It might have been a strength or power limit, or it might have been a cardiorespiratory limit. What is important is that you cannot get another set done. The only way you can finish another set is if you get under that limit again. How might you go about doing this? Decrease the intensity.

You have tons of options for decreasing the intensity. You can decrease the load. You can increase the rest time. You can perform the front squats through a lesser range of motion. You can perform fewer repetitions. You can switch to back squats. Cut back on one of the intensity factors, and you will have a chance to get under the capacity limit and continue training. A *workout dependent tradeoff* is made in response to a limit that arises during a workout.

Capacity Limits and the Tradeoff Concept

There is another kind of tradeoff known as a *workout independent tradeoff*. What makes these tradeoffs independent is that they are made *proactively* (before going into a workout) rather than *reactively* (during, or in response to, a workout). For example, imagine wanting to incorporate a bench press exercise into your program. Let's say your capacity limit for bench press is 4 reps at 225 pounds or 10 reps at 205 pounds. There is a tradeoff between strength and ability to reproduce that strength, but the decision to perform one scheme or the other does not occur during a workout in response to training. In one case, 20 more pounds could be pressed but for six less reps. In the other case, 20 less pounds could be pressed but for six more reps. What tradeoff you ultimately choose to make should coincide with your current workout, training program, and training goal. The decision is made before heading to the gym and may allow for only minor fluctuations in absolute intensity.

Independent tradeoffs will play a big role in the remainder of this book.

Now is probably the best time to discuss the role of muscle mass in fat loss. Muscle mass is sort of a pseudo intensity factor. Everyone knows that bigger muscles have a greater potential for force production. Everyone also knows that muscle mass burns more calories at rest than fat mass. Finally, everybody knows that people can train specifically to increase their muscle mass (hypertrophy training). An increase in muscle mass usually means an increase in intensity capacity.

The reason that muscle mass is not an actual intensity factor is that it cannot be modified during a workout. A person can decide whether to put 45 pounds on a bar or 15 pounds on a bar, and a person can decide how hard to train, but a person cannot decide to have 100 pounds of muscle mass during one exercise and 40 pounds of muscle mass for another exercise. It is modifiable long term, of course, but not during an individual workout.

It is easy to conceive that muscle mass can be a limiting factor, however. It is much easier for people with a lot of muscle to burn fat. It is much harder for people with little muscle mass to burn fat. Therefore, muscle mass can be a limiting factor, as a small relative muscle mass is something that inhibits one's ability to achieve a great(er) absolutely intensity.

This does have training implications, and I want to make it clear that muscle mass should be treated like an intensity factor although technically it isn't one. Much like strength training, a dedicated hypertrophy training period can be of utmost importance to a long-term fat loss program. This is especially true for those people that are training purely for vanity, because, well, muscle is sexy.

A few misconceptions need to be cleared up when it comes to hypertrophy training. Fitness professionals don't really need to read this because they already know what I'm about to say. Everyone else (especially women) needs to read this.

1. Strength training and hypertrophy training are not the same thing. I have seen a girl that weighed less than 100 pounds deadlift over 300 pounds. I have seen a guy that weighed less than 200 pounds deadlift over 650 pounds. Neither of them are huge. While muscle size is correlated with strength, they aren't the same. The methods to increase maximum strength and the methods to increase size are completely different. Big does not necessarily mean strong, and strong does not necessarily mean big.

2. Being big and being muscle bound are not the same thing. Muscle imbalances, poor posture, and inadequate mobility training are the real reasons why people lose their mobility. Size is rarely the culprit. There is a point when size will have an impact on mobility, but very few (and I mean VERY few) will ever reach that point.

3. Hypertrophy training will not turn women into hulking monsters or make them look like men. Neither will strength training, resistance band training, starvation training, sun tanning, swimming, fishing, eating, or watching TV. Steroids will. Well actually, that's not true either. Steroids plus an extremely well-written hypertrophy program followed with 100% dedication MIGHT make a woman a hulking monster or look like a man. If you are one of those women who is seriously crazy and thinks a little bit of weight lifting will bulk you up, did you ever stop to think that it won't happen all of a sudden overnight? Did you ever think that if you did start putting on a lot of muscle and you didn't like having it that you could easily just STOP TRAINING? Thank you.

Chapter 12

Functional Limits

While capacity limits apply to exercises and workouts, functional limits apply to individual people. If you recall from Chapter 10, a functional limit is something that prevents a person from being able to move effectively or efficiently. Four functional limits will be described.

The first functional limit is associated with *exercise knowledge*. This is pretty simple. Imagine yourself locked in an elevator. Could you think of 100 exercises to do with just your body weight? If you were given a dumbbell set, could you create a strength training program for your 75 year old grandmother? Do you know what a kettlebell is? *Exercise knowledge* is simply knowing what options are available and when to utilize those options for optimal results.

A *knowledge limit* is reached when someone does not know what to do in a certain situation. This could be as basic as not knowing any exercises. It could be not knowing how to program exercises effectively into a workout. It could even be as complex as not knowing how to incorporate various training phases into a long term program.

You may be wondering why a knowledge limit is a functional limit and not some other kind of limit. I like to consider it a functional limit simply because if you don't know what to do, you aren't going to be moving effectively or efficiently. You will either not be moving at all or will be structuring exercises and workouts in a way that does not come anywhere near optimal efficiency. Function starts in the brain. Knowledge is power.

Coordination refers to one's ability to physically perform biomotor tasks in the way that they are meant to be performed. If you have never been in a weight room before and are performing exercises for the first time, you are going to have relatively poor coordination. Your movements will not be fluid and might seem forced. If you find yourself in a situation like this (and it might just be for one new exercise that you are trying), then you have reached a *coordination limit*.

Muscle imbalances are also a piece of the coordination limit puzzle. Almost every person you will ever meet will have some sort of muscle imbalance. Most commonly, imbalances will be found in the hip and the shoulder, but they can exist anywhere. Muscle imbalances negatively impact coordination. The key to fluid movement is recruiting the right muscles at the right time with the appropriate amount of strength.

Take quadriceps dominance as an example. A man with quadriceps dominance is going to demonstrate a faulty squat pattern where he will tend to shift his weight forward and shoot his knees way past his toes. Rather than squatting with a good hip pattern, the quad dominant person will have a movement dominated by knee flexion and extension.

As you can see, muscle imbalances play a big role in coordination. Likewise, muscle imbalances are going to be strongly correlated to faulty posture and injury, the final two functional limits.

There is a great deal of overlap among the various limits described so far. For example, if you are fatigued during a workout and have reached a cardiorespiratory or strength limit, that may also negatively impact your coordination. You will probably discover that there are many other overlapping limits as you continue reading.

The important thing to keep in mind or to figure out is what the initial limiting factor is. If you can perform squats perfectly fine when not fatigued, then you probably just need to work on increasing your intensity capacity. On the other hand, if you are new to squatting and get fatigued because your body is all over the place, you need to really focus on your coordination.

Posture can be defined as the arrangement or alignment of the head, neck, body, and limbs. Ideal posture, if there is such a thing, is far too complex a subject to describe in this book. There have been many chapters, many books, and many programs devoted to analyzing and correcting posture, so it would not make sense to try to reproduce those here. This chapter will merely introduce you to the concept of *postural limits*.

Check out "Appendix A" of this book for a short discussion on ideal posture, common postural flaws, and potential solutions to these flaws.

A *postural limit* is a skeletal alignment that restricts one's ability to move or utilize the appropriate muscles. It might be easiest to feel this rather than just read it. So, stand up, stick out your chin, and round your upper back and shoulders. While holding that position, reach your arms up. How far do they go? Now, stand up nice and tall, keep your chin back, and then bring your arms up. How much farther can you reach?

Imagine a person with a pelvis that is tilted forward (or simply a person with a big lower back arch). This person has an anterior pelvic tilt posture. This occurs when the muscles on the front of the thigh and the muscles that extend the back are short or stiff relative to the muscles on the back of the thigh and the abdominals. What often happens in this posture is that the gluteals become weak and inhibited; the femur (thigh bone) adducts and internally rotates; the ankle everts, and the foot pronates causing the arch to collapse. The person in this posture is a likely candidate for lower back pain, hamstring strains, non-contact ACL tears, knee pain, and all sorts of other fun stuff.

Got all that?

In that case, there is a postural malalignment at the hip. It could have been caused by a muscle imbalance (such as quad dominance), or it may be the cause of several muscle imbalances. What becomes restricted in an anterior pelvic tilt posture is hip function (and a bunch of other things if not corrected in a timely fashion). One's abilities to extend and externally rotate the hip are going to be decreased, and the gluteals are probably going to be useless. For practical purposes, anterior pelvic tilt is a postural limit that is going to impact a person's ability to perform certain movements appropriately. As you can see, it is also going to be a major injury risk.

Much like coordination, you might notice some overlapping limits. If posture is your primary limit, you are going to have capacity limits such as range of motion and muscle strength (if you can't recruit a muscle, it won't have very much strength), among other things.

That brings us to the final functional limit, *injury*. An injury limit occurs when someone is hurt or gets hurt and cannot perform an exercise or workout because of it. It is pretty self-explanatory. If you are injured, your ability to lose fat is going to suffer. For a discussion of how injuries occur during exercise, see "Appendix B."

Chapter 13

Knowledge Limit Tradeoffs

If you reach a knowledge limit, what tradeoffs can you take to get by it? For knowledge limits, workout independent tradeoffs are easier to describe. Imagine that you know a man who does not know a single thing about exercise who wants to go train for the first time. He knows he has limited exercise knowledge, and before he goes to the gym, he wants to have a plan of what to do. He has basically two options. First, he can buy a bunch of books and DVDs and attend seminars and educate himself on a bunch of different methods and then go test out these methods on himself and others so that he has knowledge. Second, he can "borrow" knowledge from other people. The first option takes a long time (and is actually a lifelong process if he wants to keep up with the best methods). The second option is much easier and is more suitable for someone who does not want to make a career out of training. What does it mean to "borrow" knowledge? This can mean a few things. He can talk to his friends and let them make a workout for him. He can hire a trainer to give him a workout, or he can find a "done for you" program in a book or on the internet to follow. None of those options require that he actually be proficient at anything other than following directions.

Both education and "borrowing" can be done at the same time. Sometimes "borrowing" is a way of educating oneself. I freely admit that I have limited exercise knowledge in fields such as powerlifting, bodybuilding, and sprinting. If I had a client who was interested in any of those things, it wouldn't be in that person's best interest for me to create my own program. What I would do is find a reputable coach and "borrow" a proven program from him or her. Of course, I would tweak that program to my liking and philosophy and then be good to go. While carrying out the program, I would obviously be learning a great deal so that my knowledge would be increased and I wouldn't have those same limitations that I had before. Why reinvent the wheel?

Workout dependent tradeoffs, when it comes to knowledge, are a bit tricky. These tradeoffs need to be made when a knowledge limit is reached in the middle of a workout. What do you do when the gym is really crowded and you cannot use the equipment you want? What happens if you hurt yourself during a lift? If you do not already have a good deal of exercise knowledge, you may just be S.O.L. The tradeoff you choose might just be waiting around for your situation to improve. At the very best, you can ask someone for help. If you are gym savvy, you will not likely be in a situation where a knowledge limit is reached in the middle of training.

Knowledge goes into just about every aspect of long term and short term training. Think about it this way. If you reach a limit in any aspect of training other than knowledge, you can get back under that limit provided you have the knowledge of how to get back under it. If you are aware of your limits before you head to the gym, you can program yourself around those limits if you have the right knowledge to do so. If not, "borrow" some knowledge or educate yourself. Buy and read a lot of books. Attend clinics. Get a gym partner. Hire a fitness professional. It just might be the most important thing you can do to set yourself up for success.

Chapter 14

Coordination Limit Tradeoffs

Coordination is paramount to successful exercise. If you cannot perform exercises properly, you are not going to see results and are likely going to end up injured. The theme of this book is to constantly strive to improve in the long term. This chapter really does not need to be longer than a paragraph. It can end with the following message: practice. Practice, practice, practice. How do you become more coordinated? Practice. How do you get better at anything? Practice. How do you make it to Carnegie Hall? Exactly.

> "Not a game. Not a game. Not a game. We talkin' 'bout practice."
> -A.I.

Of course, this chapter will not end so abruptly. In fantasy land, everybody has all the time in the world to be perfect at everything. In the real world, there are coordination limits that do not have solutions that fit within one's abilities or timeframe. When these limits are identified, what tradeoffs are available?

Workout dependent tradeoffs, when it comes to coordination, are multi-faceted. Is coordination truly the limit, or is it something else? Coordination can break down when the load is too heavy or when you get tired. If that is the case, the tradeoff is resting or decreasing the load. Sometimes, coordination is the primary limit. If you are trying an exercise for the first time, it might be awkward. You might lose your balance or take a long time to perform the exercise. The tradeoff here is time. Time needs to be spent learning the exercise before it can be progressed. Maybe the exercise is not new and you have just never been able to do it. The tradeoff you might need to take is switching to a different exercise that is less intense that you can perform. Even if you think that an exercise would be the perfect exercise for you to burn fat (see chapter 6 on exercise selection), it might not be so perfect if you are unable to actually do it. Switch to a regression that theoretically is not as effective but is in practicality.

The workout independent tradeoffs for coordination limits are quite similar. If you know ahead of time what exercises you are good at and bad at, pick the ones that you are good at or spend time practicing the ones that you are not so good at.

> Random person: Can I save myself the trouble of poor coordination by just using machines?
> Me: Yes. You can. It would be stupid, but you can do it.
> Random person: Why is it stupid? It's safer.
> Me: *Blasts air horn in ears and goes to happy place*

Nothing bothers me more than people using fixed range of motion equipment that provides external stability because they claim "safety." I just don't see what's so safe about random force generation without any concept of body awareness. It has so little carry over to the real world. It trains your nervous system to produce force in aberrant patterns without simultaneously producing stability in other joints. When you try to move something heavy in a real life situation, guess what? Your back gives out because it doesn't know what to do.

Additionally, no machine fits a person exactly, and your joints are put in compromising positions. Did you know that a leg extension with 45 pounds on it puts more stress on your knee joint than performing a 200 pound squat? Did you know that a leg press puts more stress on your spine than a deadlift? So much more could be said about machine training and safety, but I will spare you the details.

What might be more important to you is whether machines are better for fat loss. As you know from reading Unit 1, the most effective fat loss workouts are those that are the most absolutely intense. How do machines compare to free movements in this manner? Let's examine the intensity factors.

The intensity factors that are irrelevant here are workout duration and rest time. You can train and rest as long as you want whether you're using machines or free weights. Moving on...

What about strength? Well, since movements are isolated, it is possible to increase the load to near maximum muscle capacity on a machine. But, do you remember the discussion from Chapter 6 about prime movers and stabilizers? How much total body strength goes into a machine workout? I'd venture to say that the strength required to use a machine is less than it is for a comparable free movement.

For range of motion, I think it is pretty obvious that machines lose. What about power? Surely you can produce a great deal of power while using a machine. However, I bet you could produce a lot more total body power sprinting, jumping, or performing an Olympic lift. Again, free movements win.

With free movements, you spend more time under tension. With a machine, you get to take mini-breaks when the machine ROM ends in a resting position. In real life, you still need to be carrying a weight. What about exercise selection? I've never seen a very complex machine exercise. You are unable to perform compound lifts and complexes with a machine. You are terribly limited in your ability to choose intense exercises on machines, so once again, free movements win.

Putting all that together, it is pretty obvious that cardiovascular load and relative intensity are much greater with free movements as well. So, why use machines for fat loss? I have no idea.

Chapter 15

Postural and Injury Limit Tradeoffs

The great thing about posture is that unless you are unaware of your own postural limitations before a training session there really should not be any workout dependent tradeoffs. Poor posture cannot really spring up out of the blue, can it? This simplifies things because you only potentially need to make independent tradeoffs. Of course, over a long period of time, posture can start to degrade as a result of poor training habits or lifestyle practices. So, a postural limit can creep up on you and manifest itself during a training session.

The tradeoffs for postural limits are time and exercise selection. Time is a tradeoff if you want to fix your posture. It is impossible to fix your posture in a single day, but it is entirely possible to fix your posture if you take the necessary steps over the course of a few weeks or months. The other tradeoff, exercise selection, is a way to avoid exercises that are limited by poor posture. If you cannot lift your arms overhead for example, you should avoid attempting to perform overhead exercises like the shoulder press. A great idea is to take both tradeoffs at once. Who says that you cannot work on correcting a postural limit while still training the rest of your body? In fact, a good exercise program should include corrective exercises that help you fix your posture.

Injury is one of those things that happens pretty regularly to people who train improperly or are simply not prepared enough to train as intensely as they try to. The best way not to be limited by injury is to avoid getting injured in the first place! (See Appendix B). Of course, that is not always possible. Does that mean that if you get injured, your fat loss program needs to take a back seat until you are healed? No, it does not. You must simply accept a tradeoff. Like postural limit tradeoffs, injury tradeoffs are usually workout independent. If you are already injured, you have options other than sitting around and doing nothing. The tradeoff you take is going to be an exercise selection tradeoff. Do not perform any exercises that aggravate the injury. Everything else is fair game. Injury tradeoffs are only dependent when you get injured during a workout.

The only thing you should do if you get injured during a workout is stop. Go home, and get it checked out. Do not risk further injury by being stubborn.

Any professional that tells you to just "rest" until you are completely healthy is ignorant or is afraid of getting sued (that, or you are really really really injured). If you hurt your shoulder, why can't you still train your legs? If you hurt your legs, you still have an upper body, right?

The first thing to do when you return from injury is take steps not to get injured again. For that, you might want to consult with a qualified professional.

Chapter 16

Time Limits and Tradeoffs

Two types of time limits exist, daily limits and global limits. A daily limit is dependent upon the day. If somebody has one hour to train on any given day, one hour is the limit for that day. Global time limits are the time limits that people set for themselves to reach a fat loss goal. For example, if somebody has to look really good for a wedding that is taking place a month from now, then one month is the global time limit. If summer is 3 months away and a girl wants to look fantastic in her bikini, then 3 months is the global time limit.

What are the tradeoffs for time limits? If a daily time limit occurs unexpectedly (something comes up during a workout) then a dependent tradeoff needs to be made. That tradeoff will usually have to be a decrease in absolute intensity (cutting the workout short, for example) or changing the planned workout in another way that skews progress towards the goal for that workout. If a person knows ahead of time what the time limit is (and this is usually the case), then the tradeoff is independent, and the program can reflect those tradeoffs. For example, if somebody is writing a fat loss workout and only has 30 minutes to train, capacity tradeoffs can be made. The load can be decreased in favor of shorter rest times, or complexes can be used instead of alternating sets. Decrease the intensity of one factor while increasing the intensity of another to save time is a fantastic tradeoff that will keep the absolute intensity at a similar level.

For global time limits, tradeoffs are independent because a long time frame will always allow proactive decision making. If a short time period is given for fat loss (say 1 month or so), then the tradeoff will have to be that that person cannot address very many limiting factors. A person with only 1 month to train does not have the time to increase intensity capacity very much or improve coordination and skill, right? So, the training program should be designed to maximize what the person already is capable of.

Chapter 17

Programming Limits

No one single program, no matter how comprehensive, will work for everyone. No program that currently exists and is yielding results will continue to yield those same results at the same rate on the same person forever. Every program, and every component of every program, for that matter, has its limits.

The important point here is that the limits of a program are 100% dependent on the level of skill, ability, and effort of the individual following the program. A poorly written program can do amazing things for an incredibly strong and athletic person with a great work ethic and the right attitude. On the other hand, a well-written program might fail someone "going through the motions." The possibilities that can be described here are endless, and it is significant to keep in mind that just because a program is not a good fit for someone right now does not mean that the program will not be a remarkable fit in a few months when other limits have been addressed.

Cookie Cutter Programs and Singular Training Modalities

1. Cookie-cutter program- any type of program where all the participant needs to do is follow along (e.g. a DVD program, exercise class, a non-customizable program from a book, etc.)
2. Singular training modality- any one type or style of training (e.g. running, dance, yoga, etc.)

Originally this comment box was going to be a stand-alone chapter designed to logically explain to you (using the theoretical model of the book) why most cookie cutter programs and singular training modalities will not work. It makes the most sense in the context of this chapter, however. So, you should use the questions in this chapter as a guide to figure out for yourself whether something is worth doing and whether it will be successful **for you**. It is much more powerful to think through something on your own than it is to read somebody else's opinion, especially when that person does not know anything about your personal limits.

Programming limits include limits in an individual exercise, an individual workout, a short-term program, and a long-term program. The following applies to just about every type of program, not just fat loss programs.

For an individual exercise, you have to ask yourself, "Is this exercise going to help me achieve my goal, and if yes, am I physically able to perform this exercise?" If the answer to both these questions is yes, then the exercise is worth programming into a training session. If not, then that exercise is limited in its worth to help you achieve your goal, and it should not be programmed. If you cannot answer these questions, then you should "borrow" some knowledge from a trusted source.

For an individual workout, the following questions must be asked:

1. Does every exercise fit the standards for being included in the workout?
2. Is the set, rep, and rest scheme aligned with the goals of this workout?
3. Is there anything else that could be included in this workout to make it more effective?
4. Is this workout compatible with daily time limits?

Again, every question should be answered with a yes for the workout to be worth doing. In regard to question 3, it is important to remember that activities to prevent injury are valuable to include in every training session. If a workout does not have an adequate warm-up, it needs to be added to the program. For more information on warming up, see Appendix C.

A short-term program will usually be written with one main goal in mind. Many different individual workouts may comprise a short-term program, and each of those workouts will have numerous exercises. That means that all of the questions from above still apply. In addition, the question that should be asked of a short-term program is this: Does this short term program provide a solution to one of the problems that needs to be addressed to achieve the ultimate goal? For example, if your ultimate goal is to lose 30 pounds in 6 months and you have a strength limit, does one of your short-term programs provide a solution to that limit?

In the context of this book, the ultimate goal of exercise is fat loss. The long-term program should thus be written specifically for fat loss. Every question already asked in this chapter should still be answered with a yes.

A discussion of programming addresses every limit described in Unit 2 and therefore provides a good summary of the unit. A program is only limited if an individual's personal limits are not addressed by the program. If a person has a low capacity limit, the program needs to address it, or it will not be effective. The same can be said about functional limits and time limits. The only question that a person needs to ask oneself for a long-term fat loss program is this: Does this program adequately address all my limits so that I can burn as much fat as possible when the time comes?

Chapter 18

Special Topic 2- Aerobics and the Energy Systems

An exercise and fat loss book would not be complete if aerobics were not mentioned at some time. The thing about aerobics is that, in general, people seem to think aerobics are a necessity when it comes to fat loss. This opinion is in stark contrast to what the general consensus among fitness professionals currently is- that aerobics are completely useless and a waste of time when it comes to fat loss.

Hopefully by the time you read this book, the opinions of both groups will have changed because I think they're both wrong!

On another note, I'd like to emphasize the difference between "cardio" and "aerobics." *Cardio* is any type of exercise that significantly raises your heart rate and keeps it up for a prolonged period of time. Essentially, any type of exercise can be considered "cardio" if it fits that requirement. *Aerobic exercise* is exercise that primarily utilizes the aerobic energy system for work periods. Circuit weight training and most forms of interval training are "cardio" but are not "aerobics."

All types of exercise use the aerobic energy system for rest and recovery periods, so just because a workout isn't "aerobic" in nature does not exclude that the aerobic energy system receives some sort of training stimulus.

To make sense of the aerobics conundrum, it is important to have a basic understanding of the energy systems. There are three: the aerobic system (which utilizes oxygen) and two anaerobic systems (which work independently of oxygen). It is important to note that all three energy systems work together at all times regardless of the activity. The first anaerobic system is the phosphagen (or the ATP-CP or alactic) system. Without boring you with details, it provides immediate energy and is the primary source of that energy at the beginning of any type of exercise for up to about 6 seconds. The second anaerobic system is the glycolytic (or lactic) system. It is the primary source of energy for activities lasting up to about two minutes. It is not quite as fast as the phosphagen system in providing energy, but it is still much faster than the aerobic (or oxidative) system.

The main reason that the aerobic system takes a while to kick in is that at the start of exercise, oxygen is not readily available in great supply to working muscles. Furthermore, the oxidative process is too slow in providing energy for high intensity activities such as sprinting. So, the only way to *directly* use aerobic exercise (such as running) for fat loss would be to exercise for long durations. Higher intensity activities (as discussed throughout this book) and time would have to be sacrificed for a lower intensity activity.

There are other drawbacks to a sole reliance of aerobic exercise for fat loss in addition to what was just mentioned. The first is that aerobic training, in the absence of other forms of training, has been shown to atrophy Type II muscle fibers. Although pounds may be coming off the scale, how can you tell whether it is fat or muscle? Losing muscle hurts a fat loss program immensely. Not only does muscle burn a significant number of calories at rest, but a decrease in muscle mass has a negative effect on strength and power, two of the most important intensity factors described in Unit 1. Second, aerobic exercise is very limited in terms of injury prevention and often contributes to many muscle imbalances, postural malalignments, and overuse injuries (See Appendix B on the mechanism of soft tissue injuries). A fat loss program should not cause more limitations!

I attended a fat loss lecture a few years ago. The presenter mentioned that a lot of his clients bring in pictures of the "ideal" body that they would like to have. (I have also found this to be true). This guy has trained thousands and thousands of people in his life, and he has NEVER had somebody bring him a picture of an elite endurance athlete (marathoner, triathlete, etc.) He said that he always gets pictures of sprinters, runningbacks, and other athletes that train for strength and power because they always have the best physiques. They have the most muscle and the least fat. Yet, sometimes his clients question his methods of training because he has them do little to no aerobic training. His response, "Oh, I didn't know you were going for the 'emaciated' look."

With all that being said, you might be led to think that aerobics have no use in a fat loss program. If you thought that (like this author once did), you would be wrong. Why? The main reason is that aerobic training is one of the simplest methods of training to program and implement for cardiac output development.

There are several other reasons why aerobic training could be directly or indirectly useful for fat loss, but to go into the details of those reasons and the methods of training would take an entire book in itself, and I probably wouldn't be qualified to write that book. (For example, I am aware that many bodybuilders stop doing high intensity interval training in favor of steady state work once they get to a certain body fat percentage.) So, for the time being, let's just stick with cardiac output development.

Cardiac output development (COD) training is something everybody is probably already somewhat familiar with on a basic level. Essentially, this method of training is meant to increase the strength of the heart muscle so that more blood and oxygen can be pumped to the body per beat. The benefits of having a strong heart are increased delivery of oxygen to working muscles, an enhanced recovery between work sets during a training session, and a possible enhanced recovery between training sessions.

Increased oxygen delivery to working muscles is important because it enhances the aerobic energy system's contribution to energy production during an exercise. An increased aerobic contribution means that anaerobic endurance will be extended (the energy substrates needed for the anaerobic systems to produce energy will not be exhausted as quickly). That means that more sets and more reps at a higher intensity can be performed before fatigue sets in, and you know by now that intensity is the key to fat loss.

An enhanced recovery during a workout allows a person to take less rest time between sets, which, if you remember from Chapter 5, is one way to increase the intensity of a workout. The other benefit is that more work can fit into a given time period, so if there are daily time limitations, an improved recovery time allows for an increased training density (intensity per unit time). Enhanced recovery between training sessions is important for a couple reasons as well. More workouts can be fit in during the week if recovery is optimized, and the injury rate is likely to be diminished for an aptly recovered body.

Cardiac output development is not necessary for all people, however. If you are a healthy individual without any known medical issues, you can easily tell if you would benefit from COD training by taking your resting heart rate. A resting heart rate of less than 60 is excellent. Less than 70 is good. A person with a resting rate greater than 70 would likely benefit from COD training.

The methods of COD training are simple to understand. All that needs to happen is that one's heart rate during exercise should remain elevated between about 120-150 beats per minute for a minimum of 20 minutes. As mentioned earlier in this book, any type of "cardio" will work. Light circuit training is fine. Performing 20 minutes of dynamic mobility work would do. There are many options. The simplest method for COD training, however, is light aerobic exercise.

Many people would want to argue with me that performing several sessions of aerobic exercise a week is going to make them small and weak and sap all their power. That is only true if you stop all other forms of training! The other argument people would have is that aerobic training is counterproductive to strength and power training because the research has demonstrated that gains in strength and power are hindered when also training aerobically. There are a few

Special Topic 2- Aerobics and the Energy Systems

questions I have about these studies. First, what is the purpose of the aerobic training? Second, how much strength training is being performed? Third, what are the methods of strength training? To have a study, there need to be controls and results that are easily measurable. The easiest way to measure strength while respecting the need for controls is to use muscle isolation machines such as the knee extension and simple set/rep schemes like 3x10.

I don't see any possible problem with this, do you? Oh wait... NOBODY strength trains like that! Also, if the purpose of the aerobic training is to improve VO_2 max (aka maximal oxygen uptake or aerobic capacity) as it is in most studies, then that style of training is far different from the style needed to train for COD! Studies are far too limited in their practical applications, and research is always years behind best practice methods.

Of course, I will not say with 100% certainty that aerobic training is not going to hinder strength and power development at all. If you are personally worried about this or upset that I would ever suggest aerobic training, then don't train aerobically! Use another exercise method for COD training. It's that easy.

Part 2: Fat Loss Practical

Part 2 will explore fat loss from a more practical standpoint than the theoretical approach from Part 1

Unit 3: The Construct Compound

Unit 3 will define *The Theory of Fat Loss* in terms
of the two constructs and will expand upon
the idea with practical examples

Chapter 19

The Theory of Fat Loss

The Theory of Fat Loss is composed of two constructs, *the theory of absolute intensity* and *the limiting factor theory*. It is probably safe to assume that if you are reading this chapter, then you have already been briefed about those two constructs. Here is a quick review for you:

1. The Theory of Absolute Intensity: the greater the absolute intensity one can achieve with training, the greater the fat loss result will be

2. The Limiting Factor Theory: within any fat loss program exist multiple potential limits that can inhibit one's ability to achieve success

3. Absolute intensity can be objectively measured with the intensity factors: strength, range of motion, power, duration, time under tension, rest time, exercise selection, cardiovascular load, and relative intensity.

4. A limit is anything that negatively impacts one's ability to achieve or maintain a great(er) absolute intensity. The limits include: capacity limits, functional limits, time limits, and programming limits.

5. When a limit is identified or reached, a tradeoff must be made. A workout dependent tradeoff is made during a workout and usually results in a decrease in the absolute intensity of that workout. A workout independent tradeoff is made proactively and may allow for little change to absolute intensity.

If all that does not sound familiar to you, you clearly just opened to this page and started reading from here. Otherwise, you are finally ready for the *Theory of Fat Loss*.

The Theory of Fat Loss states that *the greatest possible fat loss is achieved when maximizing the absolute intensity one can reach with respect to all individual limits.*

What does "with respect to all individual limits" mean? It's simple. When you reach or identify a limit, you have three options. You can *break through* the limit, *bypass* the limit, or *accept* the limit.

To *break through* a limit means that you take a "nothing can stop me" attitude. If you have a capacity limit, you break through by increasing your intensity capacity. If you have a functional limit, you break through by improving your function. Breaking through a limit requires a significant time commitment (time is the tradeoff). In certain cases, breaking through is not possible. If you have a strength limitation and only one month to lose fat, for example, breaking through that strength limit probably is not the best solution.

In these types of cases, your best option will be to *bypass* the limit. To *bypass* a limit means to avoid it entirely. For example, if you are limited by strength, you can bypass that limit by increasing your intensity by means of other intensity factors. If you are limited by coordination, you can bypass that limit by picking exercises that require less coordination. If you have a global time limit, you can bypass it by training longer and harder every day. Bypassing is a valid short-term solution to limits, but it should only be used when there are significant time restrictions. Breaking through is always better in the long-term, as it allows for more intense programming options.

Breaking through is the same exact thing as reaching a short term goal. If you decide completing 50 consecutive pushups is necessary to help you reach your long term goal, and you can only do 10 right now, then you have "broken through" when you can complete 50 pushups.

Accepting a limit means *refusing to believe that there is anything that can be done about it*. Accepting a limit is the pessimist's approach to training. In almost every situation out there, some kind of tradeoff can be made. The tradeoff may not be popular, but it may be necessary to reach a goal. It is only when all possible tradeoffs are exhausted that accepting a limit becomes reasonable.

Chapter 20

Fat Loss Programming System

As a general rule of thumb, a training phase (a short-term program written for one specific short-term goal) should last around 4-6 weeks (and probably should not last longer than 8 weeks), and then a new phase should begin. A single capacity limit can usually be broken through in one or two phases. Of course, it is definitely possible to break through multiple limits during one phase (although it is usually ideal to focus all your efforts on one major goal at a time. For example, you would not want to try to train for strength and hypertrophy at the same time. The training methods are not very compatible, and you will probably end up with inferior results than if you hit both separately). Most functional limits can be broken through during any training phase no matter what the program is designed for as long as a good individualized warm-up is a regular part of one's routine (see Appendix C). One other thing to mention is that breaking through a limit can be viewed differently by different people. For example, Johnny might decide that breaking through his capacity limit means improving his squat to 400 pounds, and Mary might decide that breaking through her capacity limit means improving her squat to 135 pounds for 5 sets of 10.

Your short term "break through" goals must be realistic. If your idea of breaking through is being able to squat 400 pounds after an 8-week strength phase, but you can only squat 135 pounds right now, then you are going to be disappointed. The solution to this is setting up multiple checkpoints. Squatting 200 pounds might be reasonable after 8 weeks, so make that your first "break through" checkpoint. Then, if you want to continue training for strength, set up another "break through" checkpoint, and then get started on another training phase. Every short term goal (or checkpoint) you set should be achievable in the time period of one or two training phases. The form in Chapter 20 actually takes out the guesswork for this process, so feel free to use it as a guide.

With this rule of thumb in mind, the first step to take when thinking about long-term programming for fat loss is to consider how much time you have available. If you have 3 months, for example, then how many phases can you complete, and how many limits can you break through before getting to that dedicated fat loss program that maxes out your intensity capacity?

Step two is to identify your functional limits. Functional limits (namely coordination, posture, and injury), as mentioned earlier, can usually be broken through at any time during any type of program with the proper warm-up. This means that you do not necessarily need to spend a month dedicated only to improving function (unless you have major limitations, in which case I'd recommend seeing a professional). Rather, you can train to break through a capacity limit while simultaneously working on your functional limits.

Here is an example if this is unclear. Imagine you have rounded shoulders and are also relatively weak. The limit that your program should address is weakness. Your warm-up can address a lot of your postural limits, and your workouts can address both weakness and posture. One of the keys to fixing your posture is strengthening the right muscle groups; in doing so, you are also increasing your strength capacity. Just avoid exercises that would contribute to the problem. (See Appendix A for a brief discussion of posture).

The problem with this step is that the less you exercise and the less you know about exercise, the more functional limits you have and the less you realize it or are willing to admit it. This causes quite an issue practically, doesn't it? It is easy for me to say, "identify your functional limits." It is difficult when it comes to actually doing it. I have met very few people (and unfortunately that includes a lot of "personal trainers" and even physical therapists) who can perform anything that mildly resembles a decent bodyweight squat or pushup, but I have met a lot of people who, when asked if they know how to squat or do a pushup, immediately say "yes" or are insulted that I even asked. Of course, when I ask these people to demonstrate the exercise, they prove to me otherwise. Luckily for all of you, I have included in Appendices A, B, and C some general tips on posture, injury, and warming up that have the potential to help you break through many of your functional limits without you even necessarily knowing that they exist.

If you get frequent muscle or joint aches or have to take time off from training due to pain or injury, or if you cannot perform certain exercises due to pain or injury, then you likely have limited coordination (which includes muscle imbalances) or poor posture, no matter what your ego tells you or no matter how much training "experience" you have. You probably could use a lot of work, and you should have someone evaluate your exercise form, especially in lifts that are causing you problems. Anyway, always warm up, return to basic lifts, fix your problems, and then watch your ability shoot through the roof. I really haven't met anybody who couldn't use more corrective work up front. It helps so much in the long run.

The third step is identifying your capacity limits (feel free to include muscle mass here as a limit). If you have any training experience at all, then this should not be a problem. (Of course, if you have no training experience, you can probably assume you are limited in everything). Are you the type of person that loses your breath walking up a flight of stairs? If so, you probably have serious cardiorespiratory limits. You know all those exercises you hate? You probably hate them because they are difficult to do and showcase your strength limitations.

The form that you can fill out in the next chapter will have a list of basic exercise categories and some value-based guidelines to help you determine what your strength limits are, so don't worry about objectively evaluating yourself without any guidance. Just use the form. Really strong people might complain that the values are too low, but remember that this is a fat loss book, not a strength training or powerlifting book. I have found these values to be fairly useful when designing fat loss programming. You don't need to be able to squat or deadlift 500 pounds or bench 350 to get good fat loss results. Of course, if you can, well then you should be able to cut fat like crazy provided you take care of your other limits!

Do not be discouraged if the strength values in the chart are much higher than your current capabilities, even in the lowest limit categories. The goal is to always improve your weaknesses as much as you can, not to be the best at everything. That is simply not always possible. Besides, even if you find yourself with major strength limitations when you need to start a dedicated fat loss phase, there are plenty of tradeoffs to choose from to maximize your intensity. The case study coming up in Chapter 23 will help clarify this. Remember, strength is only one of nine intensity factors, and, as important as it may be, it is not the end of the world if you are limited by it.

Step four is to frame your long term fat loss plan. You have all the important limits identified. Now you must decide how to train with respect to those limits. Which limits are the most important to break through in your timeframe? Which limits should you bypass?

In general, function (especially coordination) is something that is improved over time with the appropriate program. With coordination, if you have a decently long time limit, you can take your time progressing to or learning more complex or intense exercises while working on breaking through capacity limits. However, if time is short, bypassing coordination limits is probably the best option.

When it comes to capacity limits, this author believes that strength is the single most important intensity factor because of the way it affects everything else. Therefore, a significant amount of time should be spent breaking through strength limits provided the time limits allow for it. Strength probably takes the longest to increase (with the possible exception of muscle mass), which might be an issue for shorter time limits, but the good news is that strength sticks around for quite a while during periods of detraining. Cardiorespiratory improvements and local muscular endurance improvements, on the other hand, tend to disappear rapidly during detraining. With that in mind, long term programming for fat loss should focus on strength first, hypertrophy next (although these two can be interchangeable depending on the individual), and then local muscular endurance and cardiorespiratory endurance (or conditioning, as some may call it) as the time limit nears.

Before someone decides that I have my priorities mixed up, I want to point out that it is possible to blend strength training with conditioning... and so on and so forth. Creative programming exists everywhere, and I am not going to say something is not possible. All I am trying to say is that the further away people are from their time limits, the less focused they should be on fat loss training and the more focused they should be on improving their weaknesses. Furthermore, there is a hierarchy of priorities depending on those time limits. What I am not saying is that somebody can only do strength training and not burn any fat at all while doing that training. I am also not saying that it is impossible to strength train and improve cardiorespiratory endurance. In fact, with some of my clients, I will employ a strength circuit where I pick a few exercises, load them up heavily (low rep maximums), and have my clients go through and do 3-5 reps at each exercise without taking any rest and then repeating the circuit several times. Try telling me that wouldn't be a great cardio workout or that it wouldn't improve their strength capacities!

Take away point: One's primary objective changes depending on time limits, but secondary objectives are achievable while chasing a primary objective.

The fifth step is to come up with and complete your next training program/phase. What is the first limit you decided to break through when you completed step four? That should be the limit you go after when deciding upon what you are going to do in the gym for this phase. If you are an experienced gym-goer AND can look at your training objectively, then you might decide to write your own program. This has the benefit of possibly being completely individualized to your needs. It might be a good idea for you to review Chapter 17 for programming guidance. The main problem with self-programming is that it is exceedingly difficult to objectively program for oneself. So, it might be best to "borrow" a program from somewhere else that was designed specifically for the goal you have in mind. Be cognizant of your daily time limits when considering a program. Minor modifications can be made to a borrowed program based on the equipment you have available or on your own personal needs; however, it is not recommended to make major changes.

Step six is to reevaluate. After you finish your first training phase, simply go through steps one through five again. You should have different limits now. Perhaps you are stronger, more coordinated, have better posture, etc. This should help you reevaluate where you are and how far you still need to go. Maybe your first phase was not as successful as you thought it would be because of program limitations, and you need to try breaking through the same limit with another program. That is fine. Just figure out how it fits into your new time limit.

It is nice to have everything all in one place. So, in summary, your fat loss programming system consists of 6 steps.

1. Identify your global time limit.
2. Identify your functional limits.
3. Identify your capacity limits.
4. Frame your long term fat loss plan with respect to your limits.
5. Create and complete your next training phase.
6. Reevaluate yourself by going through the system another time.

Chapter 21

Assessment and Programming Forms

The following pages have a form that takes you through the *Theory of Fat Loss* programming system. You or a qualified fitness professional can use it to assess your limits and write you a fat loss program.

Printable copies of this form can be found under the "Buyer's Bonuses" tab at:

> http://thetheoryoffatloss.blogspot.com

The Theory of Fat Loss Assessment and Programming Form

Name: _____

Current weight: ____　　　　　　　　OR　　　　　　　　Current Fat Mass: ____
Ideal weight: ____　　　　　　　　　OR　　　　　　　　Ideal Fat Mass: ____

Step 1: Identify Global Time Limits

How long do you have until you need to achieve your fat loss goal? _____

Step 2: Identify Functional Limits

Coordination (choose one):

__ I have very limited training experience or ability to correctly perform basic lifts
__ I can perform basic multi-joint exercises without limit (squats, deadlifts, lunges, pushups, rows, etc.)
__ I can perform advanced lifts without limit (complexes, Olympic lifts, combination exercises, etc.)

Posture:

Write down any postural limits you have. If you do not know much about posture, see Appendix A for a quick reference to common postural problems or consult a qualified professional.

_____
_____
_____

Injury:

List any and all injuries that you currently have or that you have suffered in your life. Get evaluated by a qualified professional to avoid further injury.

_____
_____
_____

Special Notes on Functional Limits:
Examples: What exercises am I not capable of doing because of these limits? What stretches and corrective exercises should I include in my warm-up to break through these limits? What exercises should I perform during my workout to break through these limits?

Step 3: Identify Capacity Limits

Strength:
Use the chart below:

Values used are for your 3 rep maximum (maximum load you can lift for 3 repetitions) and are in pounds.
Feel free to choose any exercise(s) you want to evaluate your limits as long as they fit in the right category.
Values are just a guide, and they are not universal. The greater strength you have, the lesser the limit.

Strength Limitation:

Significant	Moderate	Mild	Minor	Not Limited

Quad-Dominant Double-Leg Exercise* (Squat, Front Squat, Dumbbell Squat, etc.)

Less than 115	115-165	165-215	215-265	More than 265

Glute-Dominant Double-Leg Exercise* (Trap-Bar Deadlift, Deadlift, etc.)

Less than 135	135-185	185-235	235-285	More than 285

Single-Leg Exercise* (Split Squat, Lunge, Reverse Lunge, etc.)

Less than 45	45-75	75-105	105-135	More than 135

Upper Body Vertical Push (Dumbbell Shoulder Press, Military Press, etc.)

Less than 85	85-115	115-145	145-175	More than 175

Upper Body Vertical Pull (Bodyweight or Loaded Pullup or Chinup**, Lat Pulldown, etc.)

Less than 135	135-165	165-195	195-225	More than 225

Upper Body Horizontal Push (Dumbbell Press, Bench Press, Pushup***)

Less than 135	135-165	165-195	195-225	More than 225

Upper Body Horizontal Pull (Inverted Row, Bent-Over Row, Cable Row)

Less than 135	135-165	165-195	195-225	More than 225

*Bodyweight has a lot to do with the absolute intensity of lower body lifts.
Due to extreme bodyweight variance, the values shown only represent external loading.
**Use bodyweight to estimate load for a pullup or chinup. Add any external load to bodyweight
***The load for a pushup is about 60% bodyweight

Note: Values to determine capacity limits are the same for men and women because intensity is based on an absolute scale, not a relative scale. The organization of the chart provides you with a quick and easy way to determine possible break through values (how much you need to lift in order to get from one limit category to another limit category). A strength break through should take approximately 1 to 2 training phases. In other words, during a strength training phase or two, it should be possible to improve to a higher limit category in every one of the exercise categories in the chart above. Women, however, may find it more difficult to break through in upper body lifts due to their genetically smaller shoulder girdles.

Muscular Endurance: Muscular endurance for any given load is largely determined by absolute strength, so no separate guidelines are needed.

Muscle Mass:* Do you have limited muscle mass, or, in other words, would you like more muscle mass? _____

*Beginners generally do not see changes in muscle mass until 6-8 weeks into training. Neurological adaptations come first.

Cardiorespiratory: (choose one)
__ I find myself short of breath with even the simplest daily activities (if so, get evaluated by a doctor immediately)
__ I get extremely tired with any form of exercise (get evaluated by a doctor before beginning an exercise program)
__ I find it difficult to perform vigorous exercise or to exercise for a long period of time
__ I can perform vigorous exercise with few limitations
__ I can train hard all day every day using any training methods without breaking a sweat

Step 4: Frame your long term fat loss program with respect to your limits

How many training phases* (approximately 4-6 weeks each) can I fit in before my time limit expires? ____
*Do not forget to include deload weeks after every 1-2 phases when making this calculation.

Which limits should I take the time to break through?
_____
_____
_____

Which limits must I bypass?
_____
_____
_____

Outline Your Long Term Plan Below using the chart (as a guide) or the space below the chart (advanced programming)

*It is recommended that you break through strength and mass limits the further you are from your time limit.

	Phase 1	Phase 2	Phase 3	Phase 4	Phase 5
Duration (weeks)					
Capacity Limit to Break Through					
Functional Limit(s) to Break Through					
Dedicated Fat Loss Phase?					

Step 5: Create and complete your next training program/phase

How long will this phase last? _____

Is this a dedicated fat loss phase (fat loss is the primary objective, not strength, hypertrophy, etc.)? ___

If yes...

How many days a week can you train and how much time do you have available each day to train?

What are your current limits (refer to Steps 2 and 3), and what tradeoffs (refer to Unit 2 of *The Theory of Fat Loss* if you need assistance) are you taking to bypass them?

_____
_____
_____

If no...

What primary capacity limit are you focusing on breaking through during this phase? _____

Are there any secondary capacity limits you feel you can also work on during this phase (advanced programmers only)?

_____
_____
_____

What functional limit(s) are you trying to break through during this phase?

_____
_____
_____

How many days a week can you train and how much time do you have available each day to train?

List any other limits that you have that are going unaddressed during this training phase that might limit what you can do during this training phase (refer to Steps 2 and 3).

_____
_____
_____

Create your program based on the assessment above
                OR
Find and borrow an existing program that fits your needs

If you need help, you will find a bunch of resources under the "Resources" tab at:

                http://thetheoryoffatloss.blogspot.com

You may also go to the "Buyer's Bonuses" tab to get a bunch of FREE customizable 2x, 3x, and 4x per week training templates for breaking through various limits.

Step 6: Upon completion of a training phase, reevaluate your ability and limits by going through this form again.

Chapter 22

Special Topic 3- Women

Is it harder for women to burn fat with exercise? You may have heard this rumor before. It is true. It is undeniable that women store and retain fat more easily than men. There exist both chemical and practical explanations for it (such as the undeniable fact that women bear children). The research that is being conducted by physiologists searches for these causes.

However, a focus on this sort of research seems unnecessary for practical purposes. The research will not provide solutions for women that they can start applying right away. Instead of researching 100 reasons why women are worse at burning fat than men, why not research 100 ways women can burn just as much fat as men? Why focus on the negative?

Not only that, but the obvious answer has been ignored. **Women are not as strong as men.** That may just be the primary reason why they cannot burn as much fat with exercise. Because of this, it is even MORE important for women to strength train. Otherwise, they will just end up spinning their wheels with the same old diet and exercise routines that do not get them the results they want.

My favorite client ever (yes, I do have favorites) was a young woman who came to me to lose 20 pounds. I was in the process of developing this theory when I started working with her. Since she was completely new to exercise, I knew that her strength would increase rapidly, so I put her on a combination strength and fat loss program. She was progressing fairly nicely in the beginning, and she told me the weight was "hard" every time I moved her up. I told her it would be nice to get her up to 135 pounds on deadlifts as soon as possible but that I didn't know how long it would take. Well, during one of her workouts, she was supposed to complete her last strength set for 4 reps at 115. For some reason, she did nine... easily. Apparently she had just been lying to me (and herself) about the difficulty of her workouts.

From that point on, I *really* emphasized the strength part of her program with her lower body lifts. Her favorite thing to tell me was "Tim, I can't!" She would then always proceed to do whatever I put on the bar. After only two months of training, she got her deadlift up to 200 pounds for 4 reps. Oh... and she lost the 20 pounds.

She taught me a valuable lesson. Women think everything is heavy at first! The important thing to know is that they are far stronger than their own concept of heavy. Every time I've trained women since training her, I've increased the load in lower body lifts rapidly. Female legs get strong pretty fast. When I work with them, I am merely the medium for showing them what they are capable of.

The problem is usually intimidation. Women are "not supposed to be strong." If you are a woman, be honest with yourself; did you see the categories in the strength chart in Chapter 21 and think, "I could never be that strong. Why should I even try?" Any woman (or any person, for that matter) who refuses to be intimidated by the strength chart in Chapter 21 and views it as a challenge rather than an insurmountable obstacle will reap the rewards of long term fat loss programming. It may not be possible to get into the "not limited" category, but that is not even close to being a requirement for reaching fat loss goals. The strategy will need to change depending on your strength, but that is the only difference. The case study in the next chapter illustrates this perfectly.

Chapter 23

Case Study 3- Using the System

The system from the previous two chapters was developed through real world trial and error while this author was working with real clients. This case study will discuss in detail the actual program followed by one of those clients and the modifications made to it that made it more suitable for fat loss. The discussion should serve as an example of how the fat loss programming system can be used.

Katie started training approximately six months before she was to attend a wedding (Step 1). She had not seriously trained in quite some time, and upon her assessment, the following functional limitations were found (Step 2):

Coordination:
Difficulty performing bodyweight squats, lunge variations, and pushups with good form
Poor motor control of the gluteus maximus and medius

Posture:
Anterior pelvic tilt
Rounded shoulders
Left shoulder carried higher than right
Forward head
Inward-facing patellas

Injury:
History of knee pain
Occasional shoulder pain

Assessment of her capacity limits (Step 3) revealed *significant* (see assessment form) strength limitations for every exercise category; she was especially limited in the upper body categories. Katie also had muscle mass limitations. She fell into the middle category for cardiorespiratory limits.

Her long term program outline (Step 4) is below:

	Phase 1	Phase 2	Phase 3	Phase 4	Phase 5
Duration (weeks)	4 weeks	4 weeks	6 weeks	3 weeks	3 weeks
Capacity Limit to Break Through	Strength	Strength	Strengh, Mass*	N/A	N/A
Functional Limit(s) to Break Through	Post, Coord.	Post, Coord.	Coord.	N/A	N/A
Dedicated Fat Loss	No	No	No	Yes	Yes

*Lower body strength training, upper body hypertrophy training

Note: If you add up the weeks, it does not equal 6 months. If you consider deload weeks, that is where you will find your lost time. Also, this is what her program breakdown looked like after we were done training, so this outline was made retrospectively, not prospectively.

For Step 5, all you need to know about the first three phases is that they ended up being dedicated to breaking through strength limits (and a little time was dedicated to upper body hypertrophy). Also, Katie's posture improved to where she had insignificant limits, and her coordination DRASTICALLY improved so that she could handle several advanced lifts. She also never suffered an injury, and her previous aches and pains cleared up nicely.

So, upon reevaluation before beginning Phase 4, Katie essentially eliminated her functional limits and improved her intensity capacity by breaking through several strength limits, putting on a little bit of muscle mass, and breaking through to the next cardiorespiratory limit (just by nature of her training). At this point, she had approximately 6 weeks left to train for fat loss.

Despite the massive increases in her strength, Katie still found herself with *significant* strength limitations for all upper body exercises. She did, however, improve to the *moderate* category for all lower body exercises.

This is actually pretty typical for many women because they usually start off at such low levels of strength. Just so you don't think I'm a terrible trainer because I couldn't get her strong, let me list a few of her strength accomplishments between the beginning and end of her first three phases. By the way, this is one reason why keeping a training log is useful.

-Went from not being able to perform a single pushup to being able to complete 3 sets of 8
-Went from only being able to perform eccentric (lowering phase only) chin-ups to being able to perform 4 sets of 7 TRX assisted chin-ups
-Went from unable to perform a barbell shoulder press to performing 6 repetitions at 60 pounds
-Took her trap-bar deadlifts from 6 repetitions at 95 pounds for half the range of motion to 2 reps at 165 pounds for the full range of motion

-Was able to perform 8 repetitions at 200 pounds for rack pulls (a shortened range of motion deadlift variation)

Referring to Step 5 on the assessment and programming form, the questions left to answer for Katie when transitioning to a dedicated fat loss phase were how much time she had available each day and week to train and how she was going to bypass her strength limits. Katie was not limited in how frequently she could train and gave herself about an hour for each training session. So, it was decided that she would have a "two days on and one day off" training schedule.

Katie had significant upper body strength limits and moderate lower body strength limits. How were these strength limits bypassed? Well, the first tradeoff was time. To get better results, she had to take less rest time between training sessions. Training two out of every three days is pretty difficult to do for 6 weeks. The other tradeoffs are best described when you can look at her training program:

*Abbreviations: RFESS = rear foot elevated split squat; DB = dumbbell; BB = Barbell; UG = underhand grip; TRX is a piece of equipment similar to blast straps.

Workout A	Sets/Reps	Rest
A1 Trap Bar Deadlift	5+, 30 tot	0
A2 Pushup	5+, 30 tot	0
A3 TRX Row	5+, 30 tot	30
B1 TRX Side Plank	2x20s	0
B2 BB Core Anti-rotation	2x8-12	30
C1 Bike Intervals	6x20s	40

Workout B	Sets/Reps	Rest
A1 DB Squat to Push Press	2x20	0
A2 DB Stepup + Biceps Curl	2x20	60
B1 TRX Assisted Pullup	2x8-12	0
B2 Ball Leg Curl	2x8-12	60
C1 TRX Plank	2x30s	30

Workout C	Sets/Reps	Rest
A1 TRX RFESS	5+, 30 tot	0
A2 UG BB Bent-over Row	5+, 30 tot	0
A3 DB Bench Press	5+, 30 tot	30
B1 TRX Side Plank	2x20s	0
B2 BB Core Anti-rotation	2x8-12	30
C1 Bike Intervals	6x20s	40

Workout D	Sets/Reps	Rest
A1 Trap Bar Deadlift + Shrug	3x12	0
A2 Rev Lunge + DB Shd Press	3x12	60
B1 TRX Assisted Pullup	3x6-10	0
B2 Ball Leg Curl	3x6-10	60
C1 TRX Plank	2x30s	30

If you look at the workouts, you will see that Katie was able to get exercises in from every exercise category listed in the chart from the form. That was by design so that she did not develop any muscle imbalances during her fat loss training. Nothing can derail an exercise program like an injury! Also be aware that Katie did complete a comprehensive warm-up before each workout the entire 6 months she was training.

The tradeoffs taken for strength were many for Katie. If you look at workouts "A" and "C", you will notice that mini circuits were utilized. Three exercises were chosen to be completed consecutively without any rest, and then the circuit was repeated after only 30 seconds rest for the necessary sets.

The other thing you will notice is the set/rep scheme for the circuits. It says "5+, 30 tot[al]." What this means is that she was to complete at most six repetitions for each set (to ensure at least 5 sets), but she could take as many sets as she needed to get to 30 total repetitions for each exercise. This allowed for the loading to be around a 6-8 rep maximum for each exercise. As she went through the circuit multiple times and got fatigued, she became less able to get to the maximum 6 reps for each set and had to move on to the next exercise. So, at the end of 5 sets, she still would possibly have some repetitions left to complete for each exercise. This set/rep/rest circuit plan allowed her to efficiently use her strength while avoiding local muscular fatigue and simultaneously demanded a great cardiac output.

The final additional variable in workouts "A" and "C" was the bike intervals. For Katie, this involved getting on an exercise bike and riding as hard as possible for 20 seconds before relaxing for 40 seconds for a total of 6 total rounds. The strength tradeoffs taken here were increases in power, time under tension, cardiovascular load, and relative intensity.

Workouts "B" and "D" used supersets of compound exercises for a high number of repetitions with short rest intervals as the tradeoffs for strength.

Despite all these tradeoffs, it was decided after three weeks that something was not quite right with this program. The workouts were too short. The workouts did not take Katie anywhere near her cardiorespiratory limit (meaning the cardiovascular load and relative intensity needed to be increased), and the proportion of exercises that were upper body exercises was too high. Katie had *significant* strength limitations in the upper body and had far fewer strength limitations in the lower body, so more could be accomplished by increasing the volume of the lower body exercises she was performing.

So, rather than complete another three weeks on the same program, another training program was designed with the previous program's limits in mind, and another phase was begun. This program only had two separate workouts rather than four, and the total number of lower body exercises was greatly increased.

Workout A	Sets/Reps	Rest
Barbell Complex*	2 sets	60
A1 Trap Bar Deadlift	5+, 30 tot	0
A2 Pushup	5+, 40 tot	0
A3 Body Weight Split Squat	5+, 50 tot	30
B1 Side Plank	2x30s	0
B2 Jump Rope	2x60s	0
C1 Bike Intervals	6x20s	40

Workout B	Sets/Reps	Rest
A1 Rack Pull	4x6-10	0
A2 TRX Assisted Pullup	4x6-8	0
A3 Step Up + Curl + Shd Pr	4x8-12	60
B1 Goblet Squat	2x25	0
B2 Ab Wheel Rollouts	2x8	0
B3 DB Swing or Vertical Leap	2x60s	60

The barbell complex from workout "A" consisted of three exercises. The first was a hang clean to front squat to push press performed for ten repetitions. The next was a bent-over row performed for ten repetitions, and the third was a single-leg Romanian deadlift performed for five repetitions on each leg. All those were performed in sequence without putting the barbell down (the definition of a complex). The obvious tradeoff taken here was an increase in the intensity and complexity of the exercise.

The mini circuit performed after the barbell complex is similar in style to the ones from the previous phase. The difference is that the total repetitions to be completed now varied for each exercise, and rather than having one lower body lift followed by two upper body lifts, this circuit had an upper body lift sandwiched between two lower body lifts (one of which was a single leg exercise, meaning that Katie had to perform 50 total reps per leg). Again, the strength tradeoffs taken here were a short rest time, a great total number of reps, and a switch to a more absolutely intense exercise (substituting a single-leg lower body exercise for an upper body exercise). These led to a greater cardiovascular load and relative intensity.

Another change made in this program for workout "A" was the addition of jumping rope during the core training part of the workout. You can see that no rest time was taken at all between exercises "B1" and "B2." The purpose of this was to keep Katie constantly working so that her cardiovascular load would remain elevated. The interval training remained the same. The total training volume for this workout was increased from the previous phase as well.

Normally I do not like to train my clients so hard that they throw up during their workouts. However, with Katie, I was frustrated that her phase 4 programming wasn't intense enough. So, I was happy when the changes I made for phase 5 resulted in her feeling like she had to vomit during one of her workouts. She didn't throw up, by the way, so I had the dual satisfaction of knowing I pushed her to the brink and that I did not need to clean up my gym.

For workout "B," you will notice that her program included two low rest time mini-circuits and four total lower body exercises. Also, you will see that the first circuit utilizes several other tradeoffs including an exercise that allows for a high load (Katie could perform 8 repetitions at 200 pounds for rack pulls at the end of her last strength phase), a high intensity combination exercise, and a voluminous set/rep scheme.

The second circuit was meant to push her simultaneously to both her local muscular endurance limits and her cardiorespiratory limit. This circuit utilized the tradeoffs of short rest times, a high number of repetitions (25 reps of Goblet Squats per set!), and a long time under tension (60s straight of dumbbell swings per set!).

Hopefully this case study provided you with a bunch of practical examples of how you could write a solid fat loss program that bypasses your limits. With Katie, she had to bypass some major strength limitations despite spending several months breaking through those limits. So, when it came to her dedicated fat loss programming, we traded strength for several other intensity factors so that she could still train at a high absolute intensity.

The other important thing to note is that we leveraged her best qualities. She was not limited by coordination, so some very intense exercises were selected for her program. She also didn't have a small cardiorespiratory limit, so we were able to challenge her with high relative strength circuits and an extremely dense set/rest/rep scheme.

I would expect that most people who are reading this book would have a story similar to Katie's. Extremely strong individuals with small cardiorespiratory limits are not the norm in our society, although they do exist. If you are one of those few people, then your plan would be pretty straightforward. Spend a phase or two breaking through your cardiorespiratory limits and then the rest should be simple (not easy to execute... but simple in concept) because your massive strength should afford you plenty of ways to execute a dedicated fat loss program.

Chapter 24

Dedicated Fat Loss Programming

Note: If you are just flipping through this book, and this is the first chapter you decide to read, please reconsider. It either will not make any sense or will give you the wrong idea.

When it comes time to put together a dedicated fat loss program (your global time limit is expiring soon), what do you do? How do you program it? You should maximize your absolute intensity by prioritizing your strengths. Answer the question, "What are you the best at, and what are you the worst at?" The program should be based off the answer.

For most people, I am of the opinion that a dedicated fat loss program should generally not last more than two months. There are two reasons why. First, fat loss programs are extremely intense. The human body was not built to endure an all out training effort multiple times a week for months on end. Without proper recovery and a change of stimulus, people get injured. Second, when I am trying to get someone to lose a bunch of fat, I program their strengths. If this happens over a long period of time, their weaknesses are never adequately addressed and they end up even more limited than they were when they started. I'm not saying someone can't do fat loss for 3+ months. Sometimes it has to be done that way. I just would be cautious recommending it for somebody.

Say you have extremely powerful legs and extremely weak arms. Program a high volume of lower body exercises. Throw in some Olympic Lifts, some sprinting, some leaping, and some heavy deadlifts and squats. Single-leg work might be especially useful because then you have to train both legs separately. Do not ignore your upper body, but just train it when your legs are recovering from their sets.

Say you rarely get tired while training but are limited by strength. Program giant sets, circuits, and exercise complexes that maximize your time under tension and minimize your rest. When you do take rest time, make it active with some jump rope, light jogging, or mobility drills.

What if you are not very strong but are very coordinated? Pick self-limiting exercises that require intense focus and balance like Turkish get-ups, bottoms-up kettlebell presses, and off-loaded upper and lower body exercises.

What if you are strong but only know a few exercises? Program a high volume of those exercises into your program. Practice other exercises during the warm-up or between work sets.

Maybe you are horrible at all things related to exercise and your biggest strength is that you are not limited by daily time limits. If so, what is stopping you from training at a safe intensity level for 6 hours a day?

Maybe you are amazing at all things related to exercise, but you have no idea how to write your own program. Find and follow a program that you know will challenge you.

The scenarios are endless and the solutions are unlimited. Of course, in real life you will likely have more than just one strength or one limit, so you will have more options available to you. Use the intensity factors as a guide. What are you least limited by? Emphasize those strengths. What are you most limited by? Bypass those limits. That is not to say that you should not go back later and break through your limits. There is just a temporary priority shift when you have to maximize your intensity right now to reach your goal.

The goal of a fat loss workout is not so much to burn a lot of fat but to speed up metabolism. The body favors equilibrium over change, so it doesn't like when you start slimming down. In response to fat loss, your metabolism will slow down more than it should (because it wants to bring your weight back to where it was before). Any type of exercise will speed up your metabolism, but some are better than others. A "finisher" is one way to do this effectively.

A finisher is something put at the end of a workout that ensures that people around you will become exhausted just watching you do it. It is an all out effort. Obviously the ability of someone to complete any given finisher will vary depending on that person's level of conditioning, but that doesn't mean I don't have a favorite. Here it is:

Partner Resisted Sprinting (with resistance band) x 20s
Clap (Explosive) Pushups x 20s
Max Vertical Leaps x 20s
Rest up to 60s (varies by person)
Repeat up to 4 times (varies by person)

The question that always comes up after somebody completes a fat loss program is, "What's

next?" Well, my personal recommendation is that a fat loss program should be immediately followed by hypertrophy training (after a week or two of rest of course). The reason is that the best time to put on muscle is when the body hasn't quite adjusted to being smaller. As I said before, your body doesn't like change, so it will "want" to get back to a heavier weight. The good news is that I don't think it needs to be fat, so why not take that time to put on some muscle mass?

Unit 4: Nutrition and Other Factors for Fat Loss Success

Unit 4 will discuss that the non-exercise related factors that can make or break a fat loss goal

Chapter 25

Nutrition Basics

You cannot out-train a bad diet. However, a poor diet does not guarantee failure... at least not immediately. Improving your diet is a process similar to breaking through your limits. You do not need to start with the cleanest, healthiest diet in the world; you simply need to improve over time so that over the course of a few months, you are far better off than you were when you started. The nutrition chapters in this book are designed to do two things. The first is to describe clean eating in general. The second is to describe the diet modifications you should make to your clean eating program to enhance fat loss.

I am not a dietician or a nutritionist, and I am not qualified to analyze your diet or create some sort of done-for-you meal plan that you can follow. The good news is that I don't think that is even remotely necessary. Let's face it. You know what junk food is and why you should avoid it. You know that fast food is not healthy. You know that REAL foods are a healthier choice than processed foods and that soft drinks go right to your abs, thighs, and butt. Almost everybody that is trying to get rid of some fat can identify several aspects of their diets that need improvement. Use these nutrition chapters as a quick reference to help you with the big picture, not as a comprehensive guide.

When it comes to diet, two things always matter. The first is the source of the calories. The second is the number of calories. Not all calories are created equal! Different types of foods are processed by your system at different rates, stored or utilized uniquely, and have profoundly different affects on your metabolism. Getting your calories from pastries, chips, beer, soft drinks, candy, and fried chicken will probably not help you with much of anything, but getting your calories from colorful vegetables, high quality fats (fish oil, olive oil, walnuts, Omega-3 eggs, free range animal fats, etc.), and complete proteins (fish, meat, or the right combinations of vegetables) probably will help you. With that being said, consuming 8000 Calories a day, even from healthy foods, is not the way to go either!

I am not a fan of counting calories directly. To me, it almost overshadows your true long-term nutrition goal of clean eating. Not only that, but the body is not even close to 100% efficient when it comes to extracting calories from food, and the efficiency differs depending on what the food is and how much food you eat. Many calories end up in your toilet, not in your body. Now, I do recommend keeping a diet log (see Chapter 28) because you can use that to better determine if you need to eat more or less food to reach your goal.

Your nutritional goals should match your workout goals. That means that if you are in a training phase where you are trying to put on muscle mass, you probably should not be trying to cut calories no matter what your long term goal is. That is counterproductive. Having said that, it is important to know some basic nutrition fundamentals that you should always be following. Depending on your exercise program or goals, the precise details will change, but the fundamentals will remain the same. They are listed below:

1. Have a meal or snack at a minimum of every 3 hours you are awake
2. Consume a complete protein at every meal (and ideally at every snack time)
3. On average, consume **at least** one serving of fruits or vegetables every time you eat
4. When you have a choice, choose the healthier food or drink
5. **Always** eat (or drink) IMMEDIATELY after a workout
6. Consistency is more important than exact details

A more in-depth look at these fundamentals will be covered in the remaining nutrition chapters.

General vs. Specific Diets

The fundamentals listed in this chapter are what I consider to be healthy nutrition basics. They are *general* not *specific*. It is my opinion that people should do everything they can to be generalists before they try to be specialists. Clean eating and fat loss diets (or weight gain diets, etc.) are compatible but they aren't the same thing.

Like exercise, start with fundamentals, break through some bad habits (i.e. nutritional limits) by replacing them with good habits, focus on consistency, and add in layers of complexity only after you master the basics. You can't run without first learning how to stand up.

Chapter 26

Eating- When, What, Why?

Eating at a minimum of every three hours serves a few purposes. The first is improved nutrient absorption. It is easier for your body to utilize nutrients in frequent smaller doses than giant meals. The second is that eating more frequently allows for greater diet flexibility. If you want to gain size, you can eat more total food if you eat more frequently. If you want to lose fat (a good assumption if you bought this book), the thermic effect of food is your ally. Every time you eat, your metabolism increases pretty significantly. So, eating 2000 Calories over 5 meals will be better for fat loss than eating 2000 Calories over three meals. Third, eating frequently normalizes blood sugar levels and controls insulin spikes. Insulin spikes are not desirable because fluctuations in blood sugar are not conducive to fat loss or to putting on muscle mass. In the long term, insulin spikes are going to increase insulin resistance.

When it comes to fat loss, a useful rule of thumb is "never be hungry, never be full." You should never eat so little during a meal that you are still hungry, but you should never eat so much that you would not be able to eat that same amount of food the next time you eat.

The other "when" fundamental is that you must always have some sort of post-workout nutrition immediately following training. Training breaks down your muscles and depletes their energy stores. A good post-workout snack or meal will have a combination of fast-acting (high glycemic index or GI) carbohydrates and a complete protein. Your muscles are extremely sensitive to insulin following a workout, so sugar will actually go to good use rather than be stored as fat. The other thing is that you want to prevent further and unnecessary breakdown of muscle mass following a workout. A meal or recovery shake after a training session will take care of that.

When I talk about post-workout nutrition, I usually recommend one of two things. The best way to go is a recovery protein shake. There are plenty of them out there, and the best ones are usually the most expensive. Many people either cannot afford these supplements or simply do not like them. For these people, I recommend chocolate milk. One serving of chocolate milk has all the right carbohydrates and protein (and in the right ratio, about 3 or 4:1) you need for post-workout recovery. It isn't perfect, but it is cheap and, in my opinion, effective.

One point that I want to make is that you do not need to go overboard with protein immediately following a workout. One study that I came across recently suggested that you only need 6 grams of protein post-workout to counteract excessive muscle breakdown. More is not better provided that you get enough protein throughout the day.

Finally, the only time you should ever be consuming fast-acting carbs such as sugary drinks or starches when you are dedicated to fat loss is immediately following a workout. Anytime else will cause insulin spikes and increased fat storage.

Complete proteins (proteins that contain all the essential amino acids) from high quality sources should be consumed at every meal and probably during every snack time. Protein is the building block of muscle (and nearly everything else in your body), and regular consumption of protein ensures that your body will have a steady stream of amino acids available to build muscle or prevent muscle breakdown. Protein also does not cause insulin surges, which is another plus. For people that are following a vigorous and consistent training program, the protein goal should be 1g of protein per pound of lean body weight per day. Going over is fine (it is actually extremely difficult to "overdose" on protein) provided that your other nutrient requirements are still adequately met.

Fruits and non-starchy vegetables are packed full of all sorts of fantastic nutrients. They have vitamins and minerals and fiber and have slow-acting carbohydrates that do not cause massive insulin spikes. The other thing is that it is extremely hard to get too many calories when you are constantly eating fruits and vegetables. They tend to have a low energy density, meaning that they have a low number of calories per unit volume. Volume triggers your stomach and brain to say "I'm full," not calories. With all that being said, it is obvious that fruits and vegetables should be consumed regularly. If you are trying to lose fat, you might want to decrease your fruit consumption in favor of leafy green vegetables which are lower in sugar and energy density.

The remaining calories in your diet that do not come from protein sources or fruits and vegetables should come from fats and carbohydrates. Fats, in general, do not cause people to be fat or have heart disease. In fact, a diet high in Omega-3 fatty acids significantly reduces the risk of heart disease. The problem is too much of the wrong types of fats. Modern western diets are loaded with saturated fats and Omega-6 fatty acids. Ideally, a balance of all types of fats (saturated, polyunsaturated, and monounsaturated fats) should be ingested, and Omega-3s should be made a priority.

Carbohydrates are a source of energy. Whatever carbohydrates are not immediately used for energy are either used to replenish glycogen stores or are stored as fat. For fat loss diets, it is usually recommended that carbohydrates only come from non-starchy vegetables. The exception to this rule is that starches, simple sugars, and other fast-acting carbohydrates should be consumed immediately following a workout.

I must start this comment box by saying that I am a big fan of the "paleo diet." I think it is very healthy and that it gets people great results. I often recommend it to people that I train. Now on to the stuff that will make people who follow the paleo diet religiously really really mad at me...

Carbohydrates, and grains in particular, have recently gotten a really bad reputation. I think it has gone too far. Now, I do want to qualify this a little. There is plenty of evidence to suggest that ingesting a lot of carbs will make us fat and unhealthy. There are also plenty of radical and powerful case studies suggesting that grains destroy our stomachs and intestines and that removing grains from ailing people's diets makes them healthy and cures their diseases. So, there has been this recommendation that grains should be avoided like the plague and are always "bad" for you. However, I just think that this is a classic example of over-reacting in the short term. Have we not learned our lesson from the whole "low fat" debacle? (I guess we actually haven't even fully gotten over that... I still see people crucifying fat, and I still see junk foods being advertised as low fat to make it sound healthier).

Think about it this way. Were there lean, healthy, and fit people in the past that didn't restrict their carb intakes and ate plenty of grains? Yes. Are there lean, healthy, and fit people today that do the same? Yes. There is more than one way to skin a cat (or so I've heard).

I'm just looking at it from both sides. I simply don't think grain consumption is the end of the world and that it will ruin your life and health. Case studies might sound convincing and everything, but they are still individual examples that should not be extrapolated to include everybody.

Carbohydrates and grains aren't bad. They aren't anything special either. If you are somebody that is trying to lose a lot of fat, how many aspects of your diet should you shake your head at before blaming pasta and wheat bread? You certainly do not need to include grains in your diet if you don't want to, and if cutting grains out completely makes you leaner and healthier, then keep avoiding them. If you are a paleo follower, fine, but you don't have to be a missionary for the cause. It's similar to those snobby MAC people who ridicule PCs any time they can, even though the only real difference is price. You can be fit and healthy if you like eating spaghetti for dinner and cereal for breakfast too.

Too much of something is usually the problem... and if you follow the nutritional fundamentals listed in this book, it would be difficult to get too many grains. The carbohydrate and grain pendulum will swing back to moderation. Disagree? You just wait.

Chapter 27

Choosing Foods

This chapter contains information you can use to help you choose healthier foods and drinks.

Drinks:
The healthiest drinks are water and non-sweetened teas. Neither have any calories, and teas have other health benefits associated with them. Drinks with calories, such as milk, can sometimes be healthy but should probably be avoided when trying to lose fat. Soft drinks, coffee with added sugar, energy drinks, sweet tea, sports drinks, and other sugary drinks should be avoided (although after a workout they are more acceptable provided you get protein from somewhere).

How do you know if you are dehydrated? If you are thirsty, you have probably been dehydrated for a while. You need to drink something immediately. Otherwise, check the color of your urine. If it is dark or moderately yellow, you need to drink more. If it is only slightly yellow or clear, you are good.

Food:
A rule of thumb is that the less processing, the healthier the food is. Basically, if it grew in the ground naturally or ate something that grew in the ground naturally, it is probably good to eat.

Complete Protein Sources: Meat, Fish, Eggs, Dairy
Poor choices- corn or grain fed non-lean (less than 90% lean) red meats, fast food meat and fish, any fried foods, genetically engineered fish, hot dogs, American and cream cheese
Better choices- canned tuna, lean red meats (loins), turkey, baked and grilled chicken and fish, any type of eggs, cheddar cheese
Best choices- free-range birds and grass fed animal meats, tuna, salmon, halibut, tilapia, other non-predatory fish, omega-3 eggs, cottage cheese

I've heard that a good ratio of Omega-6 to Omega-3 fatty acids is somewhere around 3:1. Unfortunately, most of the fats we get from meat in the modern western diet has a ratio of 20 or 30:1. This happens because of the feed given to livestock to fatten them up. Free range and grass fed livestock, on the other hand, have plenty of Omega-3s.

One of the main benefits of Omega-3 fatty acids is their role in reducing inflammation. Not only is inflammation a direct cause of cardiovascular disease, but inflammation also slows your recovery from training and injury. Fish are loaded with Omega-3s, and the fat from fish (aka fish oil) is especially potent and healthy.

Other Fat Sources:
Poor choices- margarine, corn oil, peanut oil, most liquid vegetable oils, fried food
Better choices- butter, mixed nuts, grapeseed oil, flaxseed oil
Best choices- fish oil supplements, walnuts, avocados, olive oil, flaxseed

Fruits and Vegetables:
Poor choices- iceberg lettuce, starchy vegetables like potatoes (except post workout)
Better choices- canned fruits (no added sugar) and vegetables, 100% fruit juices, frozen vegetables
Best choices- fresh fruits and vegetables (the deeper the color and the more variety of colors you eat, the better)

Again, when attempting fat loss, it is best to stick with non-starchy vegetables and to decrease fruit consumption.

Other carbohydrate sources:
Poor choices- sugary cereals, pastries, white bread, chips, candy
Better choices- whole-grain breads and cereals, white rice, baked chips
Best choices- whole-grain pastas, wild rice, quinoa, rolled oats, Kashi cereals

If you are going for healthy eating and not fat loss, there should be no problem with ingesting carbohydrates from high quality sources throughout the day. However, if you are trying to cut fat, you might just want to stick with the non-starchy vegetables and your post-workout nutrition as your carbohydrate sources.

I always get asked about supplements. Well, there are very few supplements I recommend. After all, the best "supplement" is a good diet. That being said, here are supplements that I feel you absolutely should be taking:

1. Fish Oil- This is not negotiable; fish oil is essential for health and fat loss
2. Vitamin D- More and more research is coming out about the benefits of vitamin D and how very few people get enough of it

3. Multivitamin- This is an insurance policy; if your diet lacks something, this will take care of it

There are also a few supplements that I think are valuable but that I only recommend to certain people. These include:

1. Creatine- This is great for people trying to increase their strength or put on mass (break through some limits on the way to a dedicated fat loss program); not a substitute for good nutrition and adequate protein intake
2. Post-workout Shakes- These are simple and effective, though somewhat expensive
3. Meal Replacement Shakes- These are only recommended if getting in a good meal would be difficult (like if you are running late for work and need to have breakfast)

Chapter 28

Diet Consistency

It does not matter how good your diet plan is if you do not follow it! Similarly, if you have just an "okay" plan, you can make great strides if you simply stick with it diligently. Details are often arbitrary. The real key to any diet's success is consistency. This chapter will give you some useful tips and tricks you can use to ensure that you stick with your program.

1. Make one healthy change per week

People fail when they try to do too much too soon. It is difficult to cheat when you only have one thing to focus on. Start with something simple like taking fish oil capsules with every meal. The next week, you can start eating an apple every day with lunch or stop eating before bedtime. Do not try adding something new if you have not mastered the previous week's change. Remember, your diet does not need to become instantaneously clean over night. Take little steps and allow those little steps to become habits. Before you know it, you will be on top of a mountain.

2. Shopping

Before you shop, make a list of healthy foods that you need to stock up on for the week or month. Do not include junk food on your list. Then, simply go to the store and only buy what is on your list. If you cannot handle that and are an impulse buyer who is unable to resist buying those cookies that are on sale, send somebody else to the store with your list.

3. Planning/Cooking

The majority of fat loss training takes place in the kitchen! One of the biggest problems people have with following a diet program is that they do not want to plan or cook their meals every day. They might have all the right foods sitting right there in the pantry, but after a hard day's work, eating out just seems so much more appealing. It is quicker, easier, and often tastes better. If this sounds like familiar, you need to designate one day a week as a "planning and cooking" day. Sunday works best for most people. This is pretty simple in concept but hardly anybody does it. Spend a couple hours one day planning out your meals for the week. Then, prepare all those meals and store them in labeled containers in your fridge. Then you can just grab and go. A few hours of prep work one day will lead to convenient eating the rest of the week.

It is important to note that you should not snack on what you are cooking while you are cooking it! This is a source of excess calories that you probably don't need. A useful tip I picked up from one of my clients is to munch on some very low calorie foods such as celery sticks or carrots while you are cooking. All that chewing is going to keep your mouth occupied and prevent you from over-snacking. Not only that, but you should be trying to eat more vegetables anyway.

4. Keep water on hand at all times

Eating a small meal or snack at least every three hours (Nutrition Fundamental Number 1) will help prevent extreme hunger, but you still might find yourself getting hungry throughout the day. That is why you must always have water readily available. Many times, a glass or two of water (or hot non-sweet tea) will be just what you need to trick yourself into feeling full and prevent you from straying from your diet. Water takes up space and has no calories, plus most people are chronically dehydrated, so it is the best option for curbing hunger pangs.

5. Keep a log

This is another one of those highly effective things that people just refuse to do. Every time you eat, record what, when, and how much. It should not take more than a minute or two, and it forces you to be accountable to yourself. It is easy to make poor choices if you do not think about them and do not need to see them in writing. You can also use it as a reference to track your long term progress. You might not think you made great strides in the course of a few months, but if you see it on paper, you might realize just how much better you got, especially if you followed tip number 1. Furthermore, if you are not losing fat as quickly as you wanted, you can look back at your diet log to see what exactly the problem is and make the changes accordingly. Without a log, you cannot do any of that. It is just guesswork, which is hardly consistent.

6. Cheat

One meal every two weeks, eat as much as you want of whatever you want (preferably not before a workout). Only do this, however, if you did everything you set out to do in those previous two weeks. Use it as a reward. Additionally, there is plenty of research out there detailing how planned cheating is actually beneficial to fat loss, so why not do it?

Eating Out

A friend and former client of mine, Jake "Sausage Link" Skrabacz, a man who took his body composition from over 20% body fat to below 10% body fat (and who wrote the foreword of this book), offered the following helpful diet advice for those trying to lose fat who but who also like eating out.

A cutting phase does NOT mark the end of eating out. In fact, eating out will HELP you to remain consistent, as it makes dieting seem much less about restriction and more about learning how to adapt to culinary environments in a way that suits your goals. A few helpful tips include:

1. No bread please.

Next time you order a burger, order it wrapped in lettuce instead of a bun. Order a burrito in a bowl without the tortilla or side of chips. Get all your favorite sub ingredients over a salad instead of in a roll. This goes a long way to bring down calories and carbs.

2. What comes with that?

This is a great question to ask. Most entrees you order come with a side, and most restaurants are willing to make substitutions if you remember to smile when you inquire. Typically, your best bet will be green and steamed.

3. Investigate

It's always worth doing a little research (Google will suffice) on your favorite restaurants. You might end up surprised that a local fast food dive might just be serving some relatively high quality meat, especially the privately owned ones. How are the cows raised? How do they cook their food?

4. Weigh your options.

Choosing where to eat can also make a world of difference. This is where your new found investigations skills come in handy. Simply put, choose the restaurant where you can find the healthiest available meal.

5. Enjoy!

While you do not have to give up eating out for your sanity's sake, it is worth putting the experience into proper context. It is a luxury, so get the most out of it. You still want to cook most of your meals, so take it as a learning experience. Learn how to make your food at home more like the food at your favorite restaurant.

Chapter 29

Sleep

Get a full night's sleep every night.

I mean it. Don't even try to lie your way out of it by saying things like:

"I'm a night owl."
"I don't need to sleep as much as other people."
"I'm too busy to sleep for 8 hours a night."

There are thousands of studies on the benefits of sleep and why you need it. Sleep affects your hormones which affect your entire physiology, including you ability to burn fat.

Don't cheat yourself out of it. Enough said.

Chapter 30

Attitude and Environment

Attitude is everything. Whenever you set out to accomplish something, you have to believe that it can be done. For the most part, something only becomes "impossible" when a person has a negative attitude about it. If you say something like, "I could never lose 20 pounds," you are completely right. You will never lose 20 pounds. If you think that the program in this book just simply will not work for you, it will not work. However, if you say, "I can lose 20 pounds if I follow the system," you are already on your way towards being successful.

Of course, the right attitude is another one of those things that takes time to develop. You may have failed to lose fat many times in the past, and because of this, you might feel a little defeated. In those cases, the right attitude may simply be that you are willing to give it another shot. In those cases, your attitude should change from being egocentric ("I can't lose weight. I've failed too many times in the past.") to being about the program ("This program is a good program. It makes sense, and it should work.") Then, as you achieve little successes (see Chapter 31 on goals) along the way, your confidence will shoot up, and your attitude will become positive and will reinforce your behavior.

A client of mine once attributed his fat loss success to three things. Three percent was due to training. Seven percent was due to his diet. Ninety percent was attitude.

It has been said that you are the average of the five people you spend the most time with. This is said to be consistent across many aspects of life including how hard and how frequently you train, what you eat, your attitude towards success, your relationships, and even how much money you make. For the most part, you are who you associate with. Who do you spend the most time with? Are they naysayers? Do they tell you that you can never have a six pack? Do they tell you that lifting heavy weights is dangerous? Do they tell you that your diet is not going to work because it did not work for them? If so, then it might be difficult to succeed. When you are surrounded by unsuccessful people that are always telling you that you cannot do this or do that, you might start believing them.

Maybe you are surrounded by successful people who want to help you and do everything they can to ensure your success. They train with you and give you feedback. You share your goals and accomplishments with them. They hold you accountable when you slip up, but at the same time they encourage you to keep putting in the time. When you are surrounded by positive people that believe anything is possible, you become a positive person that believes in yourself.

Have you ever heard the saying that you rise to your level of competition? It is absolutely true, and it works in reverse as well. While writing this chapter, I remembered a Chicago Bulls basketball game from November 30th, 1995, my seventh birthday. This game stuck out to me because of how horribly frustrating it was. The Bulls entered the game with an 11-2 record and were matched up against the new expansion team, the Vancouver Grizzlies, who were 2-12 and on a 12 game losing streak.

As a 7-year old with no attention span, this game was really bothering me. It was so boring, and the Bulls were losing for most of the entire game. The Bulls were clearly the superior team (they did have Michael Jordan, the best player of all time, Scottie Pippen, the best perimeter defender of all time not named Michael Jordan, Dennis Rodman, the best rebounder of all time, and Phil Jackson, the best coach of all time), but they were playing like losers against the worst team in the league. They ended up pulling out a dramatic win behind Michael Jordan's 19 points in the final six minutes of play, but that isn't the point.

The question that I asked myself was why they were playing so poorly in the first place. I mean, they almost lost to a Grizzlies team that won 15 games that season. The Bulls, by the way, set an NBA record with 72 wins that season and won the championship. Sports psychologists call it "leveling." When a team you are playing has less skill or talent, your team's level of play tends to level out. The motivation just isn't there.

On the other hand, there is a concept called "sharpening" which means that your team's level of play is enhanced when you play highly talented or superior teams. Come playoff time that season, the Bulls clearly showed the effects of sharpening because there was a lot at stake and the teams they were playing were highly talented. The Bulls easily took care of the Heat in the first round, then handled the Knicks 4-1 in round two, and then swept the Orlando Magic, who had ousted them in the previous year. Finally, they beat the Supersonics in the Finals. It wasn't very close, as the Bulls initially took a 3-0 series lead. They were sharp indeed.

The purpose of this comment box is not to show you how big of a Bulls fan I am (okay, it partially is), but it is meant to illustrate the importance of your environment. If you are surrounded by people who don't care about their bodies, have poor diets, and are overweight, you might end up being satisfied with being just slightly healthier or thinner than them. If, on the other hand, you surrounded yourself with people who were highly motivated, trained multiple times per week with a purpose, ate cleanly, and who were in great shape, you would probably not be satisfied unless you were near the same level as them. You can call it peer pressure if you want to.

So, the takeaway point from all this is to put yourself in an environment where you have no other option than to stay sharp. Don't join a gym that has more cardio equipment and TVs than power racks because people at those gyms generally do not accomplish the types of goals you are aiming to accomplish. Don't hire a trainer that doesn't hold you accountable. Don't get a training partner that cares more about socializing than training hard. But most importantly, stop hanging out with friends that make excuses for you. You'll end up playing their game and end up nowhere.

Chapter 31

Goals

The failure to establish clearly defined goals is one of the biggest mistakes that person can make. Without goals, you are just training blindly. More importantly, goals are used for motivation, and reaching your goals ensures that you are making good progress. The system described throughout this book (specifically in Chapters 20 and 21) has been designed to outline all the short term goals for you in a stepwise fashion that makes sense in context of a long term fat loss goal. If you want to use your limits and the assessment/programming form from Chapter 21 to come up with your goals, that is perfectly acceptable.

A goal needs to hold you accountable for progress. Thus, goals should be S.M.A.R.T. A goal without these attributes is ambiguous. Ambiguous goals get ambiguous results, and that is not what you are looking for!

Specific: "I will go to the gym 3 times a week" rather than "I will train regularly"
Measurable: "I will deadlift 200 pounds" rather than "I will lift heavy weights"
Attainable/**R**ealistic: "I will lose 40 pounds in 6 months" rather than "I will lose 40 pounds in 1 month"
Timely: "I will fix my posture in 4 weeks" rather than "I will fix my posture [eventually]"

When it comes to fat loss, there are three different types of goals you should consider making: habit-based, performance-based, and outcome-based.

A habit-based goal is defined by "doing." For example, "I will train every Monday, Wednesday, and Friday for the next 4 weeks," is a habit-based goal. You reach your goal simply by following a routine. These types of goals work equally well for both diet and exercise.

A performance-based goal is defined by concrete numbers. "I will be able to perform 3 sets of

10 pushups in 4 weeks," is a performance-based goal. These goals work the best when it comes to breaking through strength limits.

An outcome-based goal is defined by the end result. "I will drop 4 dress sizes by my friend's wedding," is an outcome-based goal. Usually this type of goal is going to be the long-term goal. If you want to lose 20 pounds of fat, then this should be a part of your outcome-based goal.

Personally, I find that habit-based goals and performance-based goals are the best way to go when it comes to making short-term goals. As I've tried to make clear, consistency is the most important factor in any fat loss program. Consistency is all about habit. If you have good training and diet habits, then you will make progress. Performance-based goals are the other part of the puzzle. Even if you never miss a day on your training schedule, you will not make as much progress if you do not strive to improve your performance.

I do not find outcome-based goals to be useful as short-term goals for fat loss programs. Fat mass comes off the body at varying rates depending on the training program and diet. It can be very disappointing to set a short-term fat loss goal because the pounds may not be coming off at a consistent or linear weight. If you want to lose 15 pounds of fat in 3 months, losing 5 pounds that first month may not be a very good short-term outcome-based goal if you are strength training, but losing 15 pounds after three months would still be a fantastic long term goal.

It is important to reward yourself when you reach your goals. It is another little extra incentive to work hard. Now, it is not recommended that you reward yourself by skipping training sessions or eating poorly, but it is a good idea to do something nice for yourself. The reward does not have to come from only yourself either. Perhaps you can convince a friend to buy you something, take you somewhere, or give you a massage if you are successful. That is actually a great way to build a positive environment and get others to support you and buy into what you are doing as well!

One last thing...

Write down your goals! Post them in a place for everybody to see, and have a way to track them. Do not allow your goals to be governed by your memory. Revisionist history is not conducive to fat loss!

Conclusion

The mistake almost everybody makes when training for fat loss is having one big unrealistic expectation- that a fat loss program will yield instantaneous and long term results with only short term effort. We live in a quick fix society that is focused on the here and now. Planning and long term commitment have been lost, and that is why we fail.

Have you ever heard of *the law of the farm*, a concept from author Stephen Covey? The law of the farm teaches us that success comes to us in a fashion similar to how a harvest comes to a farmer. It would be foolish to start with the harvest because there would be no crop! For a farmer, yielding a successful crop takes preparation and dedication to a process.

First, the field must be prepared. A farmer cannot simply toss some seeds into the ground without first plowing and fertilizing the field. After the right seeds are planted, the farmer must be dedicated to tending his crops. What happens if he fails to water them, or if he does not protect them from pests? What if he over-fertilizes them? What if he under-fertilizes them? Finally, after months of care, there is the harvest. If a farmer harvests too soon, the crop will not be ready for use. If he harvests too late, the crop will be past its peak ripeness. The most important part of this long process, however, is not any individual step. It is belief in the system.

Fat loss training is much the same. There are no immediate results from exercise. It starts with preparation of the field. What limits have you identified as obstacles? What is your plan for those limits? Next you must plant the right seeds. Your seeds are capacity and function. These seeds are planted when you find the correct programs; you cannot expect to get stronger if all you do is run. The next step is tending your seeds so that they may grow. Show up for every workout. Put forth your best effort every time you set foot in the gym. If you are consistent and diligent, you will start seeing results. You reap what you sow. Finally, there comes the harvest. Your harvest is your dedicated fat loss program. If you try to complete it too soon, you will not get the results you want. If you try too late, your time limit will expire before you reach your goals. If you do it just right, you will be pleased with what you yield. Like farming, you must believe in the long term efficacy of the system, or you will get frustrated, give up, and not accomplish anything.

All analogies break down at some point, and this one is no different. Every year, a farmer must go through the entire process again. In fitness, you have the opportunity to continue growing year round. As long as you continue to train, you will never need to start back as an infant seed ever again. Success breeds success, and there is always something more to work for no matter how strong, how coordinated, or how fit you are.

In the introduction of this book, I wrote that the theory of absolute intensity and the limiting factor theory come together to create a new paradigm for exercise: the theory of fat loss. Maybe I should not have written that this theory is a new paradigm. A dedication to continuously improving ourselves and a belief that we can overcome any limits is simply a long lost paradigm that we all should bear in mind.

Upon reviewing this book before its release, a friend of mine said to me, "It's amazing how little your fat loss book is actually about fat loss." I could not agree more. Best of luck to you on your journey.

-Timothy J. Ward

The Appendices

All that extra stuff

Appendix A

Posture

"Ideal" Posture

Ideal posture is not a black and white issue, but here is a very brief description of what may be considered good posture. This is by no means a comprehensive or exhaustive description of posture.

Overall
From a side view, if a vertical line is drawn from the back of the ear to the floor, the line should go through the middle of the shoulder, through the lower back, and just in front of the knees and ankles.

Head
The back of the ear is in line with the middle of the shoulder.

Shoulders
Both shoulders are at the same height. The scapula (shoulder blade) is against the rib cage and not visible.

Thoracic Spine
The upper back has a slight convexity (backward curve).

Lumbar Spine
The lower back has a slight concavity (forward curve).

Pelvis
The pelvis is level on both sides. The belt line is level all the way around.

Knees
The knee caps point forward.

Toes
The toes do not point inwards, and they do not point outwards more than 10 degrees.

Common Postural Flaws
This is a description of common postural flaws, what might be causing them, what problems they might cause, and possible solutions. This is by no means a detailed guide towards fixing any of these problems. DO NOT perform any exercise that causes pain. Get checked out.

Forward head posture
Description- From a side view, the base of the ear is further forward than the mid-line of the shoulder
The cause- weakness of the deep neck flexors, usually from sitting at a desk all day
Problems- neck pain, limited shoulder movement
Potential Solution- static stretch the muscles of the back of the neck and perform chin tuck exercises for the deep neck flexors

Rounded shoulders and excess thoracic kyphosis
Description- from a side view, there is a big backward curve in the upper back and the shoulders are carried forward; from a rear view, the scapula (shoulder blade) is visible
The cause- prolonged sitting or time spent in front of a computer
Problems- neck or shoulder pain, inability to lift arms completely overhead, decreased shoulder external rotation, weak upper back musculature
Potential Solution- foam roll the thoracic spine to increase extensibility, foam roll and static stretch the pectoral muscles, perform exercises for the middle and lower traps, the serratus anterior, and the shoulder external rotators

Anterior pelvic tilt
Description- the arch in the lower back is excessive, the belt line is lower in the front of the body than in the back
The cause- shortness and stiffness of the hip flexors and lower back muscles relative to the glutes, hamstrings, and abdominals
Problems- low back pain, inability to properly recruit gluteal muscles, knee pain, ankle and foot pronation, makes you look fat
Potential solution- foam roll and static stretch the quadriceps and hip flexors, perform gluteus maximus (glute bridge) and medius activation exercises (side-lying clam) throughout the day, strengthen the glutes and hamstrings

Posterior pelvic tilt
Description- there is no arch in your lower back (flat back)
The cause- short and stiff glutes, hamstrings, and abs relative to the hip flexors and low back muscles
Problems- back pain, strong likelihood of disc herniation
Potential solution- foam roll the hamstrings and glutes and then static stretch them (without allowing the spine to round), place a towel roll behind your back when sitting to promote an arch, strengthen the quadriceps and lower back muscles

*For more in depth descriptions of posture and solutions to common postural flaws, check out the resources page of http://thetheoryoffatloss.blogspot.com

Appendix B

Mechanism of Soft-Tissue Injuries

The Law of Repetitive Motion
I first learned about the law of repetitive motion from two fitness professionals (Mike Robertson and Eric Cressey) and their "Building the Efficient Athlete" DVD set. The law states that

$I = NF/AR$
where
I stands for Injury to tissue
N stands for Number of repetitions
F stands for Force of each repetition **as a percentage of maximal strength**
A stands for Amplitude (aka range of motion) of each repetition
R stands for Rest (between reps, sets, training days, etc.)

This equation is similar to a mathematical formula but it is not as exact as one. It is more of a guiding equation that models a mechanism of injury. As you can see by the equation, the factors that contribute to injury are increased repetitions and increased % of maximal force output. The factors that reduce injury are increasing the range of motion of each repetition and taking adequate rest time during training and between training sessions. Also, there is a threshold. If you stay under the threshold, you will not get injured, but the further you go over the threshold, the greater the severity of the injury will be.

Basically the equation comes down to this. **People get injured if they try to do too much too soon.** Maybe they try to lift too heavy without first training to get strong. Maybe they do too many repetitions (runners are the biggest culprits of this). Maybe they push themselves too hard without resting. Maybe their form is terrible, and they did not take the time to learn how to move through a correct or a full range of motion. These all fit into that same category of too much too soon.

A few things still need to be described in a little more detail as they are not immediately obvious upon viewing the equation. Take fatigue for example. Does fatigue fit into this model as an injury factor? Yes. If you think about it carefully, can you think of what causes fatigue? High reps, high percentage of maximal force produced per repetition, and short rest time can contribute to fatigue. All three of those are accounted for in the equation.

What about faulty mechanics? Those definitely contribute to injury, but are they accounted for in the equation. If you think about faulty mechanics as muscular compensations (using the wrong muscles to "cheat" a movement pattern), then everything makes perfect sense. Inability to properly utilize the gluteal muscles is a common problem. If a person with this problem tries to participate in high intensity sporting activities, other muscles will have to produce a lot more force to take up the slack. How many athletes pull their hamstrings, strain their quadriceps, or pull their groins? The part of the equation that is being discussed here is F. When the wrong muscles are recruited, they use a much higher percentage of their maximal force capability as compensation for the under utilization of the prime movers. If F is too high for too long, injury is going to result.

One point the equation does not address is that range of motion has a limit. Obviously there exists a potential to go to far just as there is a potential to not go far enough. A full range of motion for an exercise is good. Going too far will cause muscle tears or other injuries, and not going far enough may lead to muscle imbalances. Furthermore, in some regions of the body like the lumbar spine (low back), for example, range of motion is not typically something you want to train at all.

Finally, how does soft tissue work (massage, trigger point therapy, foam rolling) fit into this equation? The purpose of soft tissue work is to improve muscle tissue quality, release areas of excess muscle tension, and to increase tissue extensibility. In other words, soft tissue work can help improve the force capabilities of muscles, improve the quality of rest time, and help correct muscle imbalances and range of motion limitations.

Practically, what can one do to decrease the risk of injury? The best options include training to increase maximal strength, taking deload weeks (time periods where intense training activities are limited) after every training phase, participating in frequent and supervised training to improve skill and coordination, and getting regular soft tissue work.

Luckily this author's interpretation of *the law of repetitive motion* and *the theory of fat loss* send the same message. Prepare.

Appendix C

The Warm-up

The purpose of a warm-up, as you have probably heard many times before, is to prepare the body for exercise. Along those same lines, you have probably heard that a warm-up increases your heart rate, increases the temperature of your muscles to help them contract, and improves your flexibility to prevent you from getting hurt. It is also likely that somebody you have come across has told you that a good warm-up only need to include some light jogging and stretching. Is any of this new? No, of course not. In fact, it is extremely old and outdated. Ask yourself this, "Are any of those facts listed above compelling enough for me to actually warm up?" No, they are not. It is no surprise that the majority of people that work out skip the warm up entirely.

A real warm-up is not limited to some light jogging and stretching. Light jogging, in most cases, is a waste of time. It is a mindless, skill-less activity with few benefits. The same goes for stretching. When most people stretch, they do it half-heartedly, and they usually stretch the wrong muscles. In the modern era of fitness and sports training, this warm-up will not cut it.

What is the real purpose of a warm-up? The many benefits of a warm-up may include, but are not limited to, the following:

1. Improving soft-tissue quality
2. Improving soft-tissue extensibility
3. Correcting muscle imbalances
4. Improving coordination and skill
5. Learning new exercises
6. Improving mobility
7. Preventing injury
8. Preparing the body for training

Not all of those necessarily need to be addressed each and every warm-up; however, at a bare minimum, the following activities should be a part of a comprehensive warm-up:

1. Soft-tissue work
2. Corrective static stretching (specific to the individual and/or the activity)
3. Dynamic mobility drills
4. Muscle activation drills

The following are additional activities that are a good idea to include in the warm-up:

1. Balance and coordination drills
2. Practice exercises
3. New exercises
4. Activity specific drills

A few more things need to be said about the warm-up. Soft-tissue work should always be completed first, and corrective static stretching should always be done immediately afterward. There is a lot of research out there saying that soft-tissue work and static stretching negatively affect performance if performed immediately before vigorous activity. However, the studies that suggest that performance is impacted demonstrate statistical significance, but do they show real world significance? Does 5% really matter in real life if it is only an inch off a vertical leap or a couple of pounds off a 1 rep maximum for a lift? Very few people reading this book are going to go out and participate competitively in sprinting or powerlifting or high jumping. Not only that, but most of these negative effects are completely canceled out by performing a dynamic warm-up. The benefits of soft-tissue work and corrective static stretching (especially if followed by a dynamic warm-up) far outweigh the potential "risks." So, grab your foam roller and get to work, and only stretch muscles that need it. It is okay to get an assessment from a qualified professional if you do not know what muscles need correction.

The order you perform dynamic mobility drills and activation drills is not very important. In fact, for advanced gym-goers, mobility drills can be combined with activation drills. How does a *high knee walk to walking spiderman with posterolateral reach* or a *pull back butt kick to cross-behind reverse lunge with reach* sound?

Anyway, mobility is important because it is "active" flexibility. Flexibility just describes the available range of motion at a joint. Mobility describes the useful, controllable range of motion available at a joint. Mobility always has context. Flexibility does not. Just because you can flex your hips to 120 degrees does not mean that you can perform a squat. Who cares if you can lick your elbow or actually put your foot in your mouth?

Muscle activation drills are also important because they can let you know whether the right muscles are working or not, and they can prime those muscles for more advanced activities that will be taking place during the workout. Most people need specific drills for their gluteal muscles, lower traps, serratus anterior, and shoulder external rotators. However, different people have different needs.

The need to add the optional warm-up activities is highly dependent upon individuals. For example, a basketball player might want to perform some agility drills during a warm-up to prepare for those types of movements during the game, and a weight-lifter might want to do some warm-up sets before loading a barbell for heavy work sets. Practice exercises allow somebody to reinforce perfect form in a de-loaded state before moving on to more loaded exercises in the workout, and new exercises can be learned and practiced in a warm-up so that time does not need to be wasted in the future when moving on to a new phase of training.

Now that you understand the purpose and the components of a warm-up, you should probably be given at least some sort of template for completing a warm-up. The following will not be comprehensive and will require that you look some things up on your own, but it is a good starting point for a beginner.

Soft-tissue Work (foam roller, tennis ball, lacrosse ball, broomstick, somebody's hand, etc.):
Upper body: thoracic spine, lats, posterior capsule, upper traps
Lower body: quads, hamstrings, adductors (inner thigh), TFL, IT band (outside of thigh), calves, foot arch

Static-stretching (30 second hold of a muscle, should not be painful): depends on the individual, see Appendix A on common postural flaws for potential solutions

Dynamic Mobility and Activation:
Upper body: focus on thoracic spine mobility (especially extension and rotation), scapular stability and upward rotation (lower traps and serratus anterior specifically), and shoulder external rotation
Lower body: focus on glute activation (glute bridges and clamshells are good starter exercises), hip mobility (especially abduction, extension, and external rotation for most people), and ankle mobility

----

This author has seen the restorative effects of a good warm-up do wonderful things for people. People who have complained about neck pain, shoulder pain, back pain, knee pain, etc. and who have believed in the system have been completely relieved of those nagging issues. Athletes who had obvious restrictions and physical limitations and who have oft been on the injured list have been freed from their proverbial shackles and have been able to show off their capabilities on the field after improving their warm-ups. These results are common. When a person goes from never performing a warm-up to including a quality one each and every training session, good things ALWAYS happen.

Appendix D

Youth Obesity

This book applies to adult populations only. While youth obesity is a prevalent societal problem, it is wrong to train kids like they are adults. It is wrong to send kids to "fat camps." It is wrong to train kids for the sole purpose of absolute muscular strength so that they can train at a greater absolute intensity. It is wrong to push kids so hard that they learn to hate physical activity. Kids simply need to enjoy living an active lifestyle. Play, fun, and socialization are important pieces of youth fitness. So are coordination and skill acquisition. While fat loss may be and often is the result of any youth fitness activity, it should NEVER be the main focus.

Have you ever heard of the Pygmalion (aka the Rosenthal) effect? In a nutshell (and without citing the hundreds of articles written about the subject), the Pygmalion effect is this: people internalize the expectations placed upon them. When kids are labeled as stupid, they tend to view themselves as stupid and get poor grades. When kids are labeled as smart, they tend to view themselves as smart and get good grades. The same goes for labeling "fat" kids. When kids are sent to "fat camps" or ridiculed, chastised, and told they need to exercise, all that does is make them internalize their "fatness." They become forever fat because that is the expectation placed upon them. It becomes a self-fulfilling prophecy. That, or they develop eating disorders. Either way, kids should not be trained because their parents think they are fat.

Every parent, teacher, and coach needs to know that kids need a variety of physical stimuli for optimal development. The more physical activity kids participate in, the better off they are, provided that the environment is positive and uplifting. This is not to say that children should not be challenged or that they should avoid getting tired and sweaty. Activity simply needs to be fun and engaging, and children should be encouraged to participate and thanked for giving forth their best effort when they do. It is the only way to go to combat youth obesity. For the best information on working with youth, check out the International Youth Conditioning Association at http://iyca.org.

Made in the USA
Charleston, SC
08 January 2011